Fat Wars

45 Days to Transform Your Body

Revised and Updated Edition

Brad J. King

MACMILLAN CANADA
TORONTO

First published in Canada in 2002 by
Macmillan Canada, an imprint of CDG Books Canada

National Library of Canada Cataloguing in Publication Data

King, Brad (Brad J.)
    Fat wars : 45 days to transform your body

Includes bibliographical references and index.
ISBN 1-55335-017-0

1. Weight loss. 2. Reducing diets. I. Title.

RM222.2.K56 2002   613.2'5   C2002-900325-3

Cover photo by David Hanover/Stone
Author photo by Scope Photography, Victoria, B.C.
Cover design by CS Richardson
Text design and typesetting by Darlene Eiler/Heidy Lawrance Associates

Macmillan Canada
An imprint of CDG Books Canada Inc.
Toronto

Printed in Canada

1 2 3 4 5 TRANS 06 05 04 03 02

Contents

FOREWORD

As a nutritional researcher with a traditional background, I have spent many years watching the successes and failures of traditional medical practices on weight loss.

The scientific approach is the right one, but researchers, authors, and health professionals must keep open minds, look at all the evidence, and be willing to change their assumptions when findings don't support them.

In this inspiring book, Brad King has compiled conclusive evidence on the benefits of adopting a new lifestyle that incorporates a dietary strategy and a sustainable exercise protocol to let you, once and for all, lose weight intelligently. Brad's approach is scientifically grounded, with a refreshing and comfortable approach that guides you step by step by step. Ancient wisdom and modern science coalesce into an easy-to-follow prescription that works. Yes, it really works!

You hold in your hands a remarkably helpful book. It will explain why many of us may be fat in the first place. It is chock-full of tips on how to incorporate proven exercise strategies and healthy eating habits into your day-to-day life that will, at long last, result in permanent fat reduction. It is the information you need to help you navigate through a sometimes confusing world where weight-loss misinformation is the rule rather than the exception.

As important as the material in this "must-read" book is, it is the enthusiasm and commitment of its researcher and writer that strike you deeply. Brad takes your hand and leads you through the land mines of confusion toward a dietary and exercise strategy that allows you to eat abundantly while spending less time exercising and lose critical pounds quickly. You may have heard this claim before. However, this book is different from any other because it approaches weight loss from a new perspective, the one that proves that not all weight is bad. *Fat Wars* is a triumph. You will not only finally be able to shed those excess pounds, but also it is likely that your life will be extended, overall health improved, energy and endurance boosted, appetite controlled, and your concepts about food and exercise radically changed for the better. A healthy diet and an exercise program are the cornerstones of a healthy lifestyle. Good food should provide pleasure and satisfaction as well as nourishment, and should support rather than undermine the body's natural healing potential. Exercise should be gratifying rather than confusing.

Look beyond the failures of your past and follow the steps as Brad guides you through. You will be thrilled by the positive results. I find this book fascinating and genuine—it adds an exciting new dimension to the real secrets of permanent fat loss.

Bravo to you, Brad King, for your diligent research and sincere dedication! Bravo to you, the reader—it is as simple as becoming aware of how you became overweight to begin with, and then taking the necessary steps to gain victory, one battle at a time. You will never regret it. The time to begin is now! Bon appétit.

I wish you abundant good health.

Sam Graci
Author, *The Power of Superfoods* and *The Food Connection*
Researcher and Formulator of greens+

ACKNOWLEDGEMENTS

I have always known that the effort we invest in our health today reaps huge dividends tomorrow. Unfortunately, many of us still believe that we are subject to whatever cards we're dealt, and that no amount of lifestyle alterations will change our bodies or our lives. (Worse, many people seem to have been dealt cards for bodies gone awry.) Research shows, though, that when it comes to obesity and its many spin-off ailments, you are the one most responsible for the outcome. If you continue to ignore this fact today, you may end up suffering tomorrow.

I have been lecturing on this preventable and reversible body transformation for many years. After my many lectures on the topic in the past, I would be approached by people asking if I would write a book on the subject. There was just too much information to explain it all in an hour-and-a-half talk. It is for these people, as well as others who are both confused and frustrated by the propaganda of the diet industry, that I finally decided to create *Fat Wars*.

Do you ever notice how many of us frenetically invest financially for our tomorrows, but how few of us are actually around when the time comes to enjoy the fruits of our labors? This book is a wake-up call to start investing in your biological future.

I owe a great debt to many people who have played an important role in shaping my destiny today and influencing the writing of this and other books. I wish to pay a special thanks to the following people.

My late mother, Elva, who unselfishly showered me with her unconditional love and the belief that I could accomplish whatever I desired. You will never be forgotten. My late father, Alan, who without realizing it, pushed me to always strive for higher ground in life.

My soul mother, Peggy Groom, who was sent from above to teach me the ways of the heart, constantly guiding me with her gentle words of wisdom. You are truly a gift from the Universe, Peggy, and I am forever grateful for you. To one of my closest friends and mentors, Sam Graci, a true humanitarian, who has always amazed me with his ability to energize those around him. You have inspired me to be the researcher, lecturer, and health advocate I am today. To my great friend and mentor, Dr. Michael Schmidt. You are one of the most humble and brilliant researchers and educators of our time. Your messages of health and wholeness are clearly needed. To Beth Potter, truly one of the best publicity agents and supporters I could ever have asked for.

To the original CDG Books Canada team for first seeing the importance of *Fat Wars*. Thanks for understanding the importance of the overall message. To Stewart Brown, for his continued support of my research. To one of my greatest supporters and best friends, Fred Hagadorn, who has always amazed me with his incredible ability to communicate with everyone around him. I have yet to catch you frowning. To Deane Parkes, my great friend and supporter, who believed in my abilities to educate others. A deep gratitude and thanks to my two beautiful sisters, Debbie and Lisa, who are always a part of my heart, whether I express it or not. To Chris, I love you like a third sister.

To Renee, my source of balance, whom I extend a very special thanks to for coming into my life. You have touched my heart with your compassion and understanding time and again, and words alone cannot express what you mean to me.

Finally, special thanks go out to all the researchers of the world who tirelessly search for new ways to battle the bulge and end the Fat Wars once and for all. This book would not be possible without all of your research to draw upon.

Health, happiness, and longevity to you all.

Brad J. King, 2002

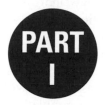

PART

I

So We're Fat.
So What?

Since you're reading this book right now, you're probably a little concerned with those additional pounds of fat you seem to have accumulated out of thin air over the last few years or so. Or perhaps you have been battling a weight problem your entire life and have run out of places to turn. Whatever the reason is, I'm glad you've picked up this book, because it's never too late to teach your body how to be healthy and lose excess body fat. But before we get into the hows of losing the fat, do you really know why it is so important to do so (beyond the cosmetic reasons)?

Everyone knows that smoking kills. Warnings against the ill effects of smoking are everywhere you look—just try to avoid them. What would you say if someone told you that it was actually more dangerous to be overweight than to be a smoker? You probably wouldn't believe them. Yet, according to a new study by the RAND Institute in Santa Monica, California, published in the British journal *Public Health in 2001*, obese adults have more chronic health problems than their smoking counterparts.

An interesting fact is that more people are overweight or obese than, *collectively*, smoke, drink heavily, or live below the federal poverty line. So you're not alone. And, in fact, it's *easy* to become over-fat. Your body naturally wants to put on weight, as I will explain in later chapters. But that doesn't mean you should shrug your shoulders and accept the extra pounds.

What you are about to read will be an eye opener, to put it mildly. These statistics are not here to scare you, but instead to make you aware of the mounting problems associated with letting our bodies go. In Canada, over 50% of our adult population is carrying too much fat. In the U.S., the numbers jump to 60% for men and women over the age of 20, with one-quarter of them being visibly and clinically obese. Each year, the problem gets worse. Canadian obesity rates have gone from 13.4% to 22.3% (an increase of more than 50%) in the last decade. Since 1991, obesity has increased throughout North America, in both genders and across all races, age groups, and educational levels. In other words, fat doesn't discriminate.

And here's the kicker: Almost 300,000 adults die throughout North America each year from conditions that are directly attributable to obesity. These are mortality figures one might expect from a major war, and they don't even take into account the myriad complications associated with excess fat accumulation.

Our ideal weight is the weight at which our risk of dying prematurely is statistically the lowest. *Obese* is usually defined as 25% or more above our ideal weight. Over-fat is somewhat less fat than that.

Establishing an ideal (and actual) weight can be exacting. However, most of us can get a ballpark figure by using a method that takes into account our height, our bone structure (fine or heavy), and how much muscle we have on our frames. Generally speaking, we know when we're carrying too much body fat. So, is this just a matter of us wearing bigger clothes? Is it just about looking bad and feeling worse? Isn't this a personal choice?

IT'S NOT ALL COSMETIC—WHY LOSING FAT MAKES SENSE

Being over-fat sets us up for a whole host of ailments, such as heart disease, diabetes, high cholesterol, high blood pressure (hypertension), stroke, cancers (gastrointestinal, prostate, breast, endometrial, etc.), gall-bladder disease, immune dysfunction, gallstones, sleep apnea and other breathing problems, infertility, osteoarthritis (degeneration of the cartilage and bone in the joints), lower back pain, complications of pregnancy, menstrual irregularities, psychological disorders such as depression, and post-surgical complications.

The number one killer in North America, cardiovascular disease, comes early to the over-fat because the blood vessels or microcapillaries simply begin to wear out faster. They can actually fail three times as quickly as they do in someone who is lean. Too much body fat (especially if the majority of that fat is located in your midsection) also greatly increases the risk of developing the prevalent condition referred to as Syndrome X, a syndrome common among sedentary, over-fat Western humans, which is strongly characterized by Type 2 diabetes, hypertension, chronically elevated triglycerides, glucose intolerance, obesity, chronically elevated cholesterol levels, low HDL cholesterol (good cholesterol), and heart disease.

Of those with diabetes, it's estimated that 85% are over-fat; many are obese. Their condition sets them up for a host of diabetes-related complications, including blindness (diabetes is the leading cause of new cases of blindness in adults), kidney failure (diabetes is the leading cause of end-stage renal disease, accounting for about 40% of new cases), heart disease (the leading cause of diabetes-related deaths), and amputations.

It is sad to think that most people headed toward these diseases would rather take numerous pharmaceutical prescriptions to keep their conditions in check than make the appropriate lifestyle changes to return themselves to a more healthful state.

Being over-fat is more than just a cosmetic issue. It's also a serious health issue, with these diseases quietly costing all of us billions of dollars each year. The direct cost of obesity in Canada has been estimated at 2.4% of the health care budget, with the three largest money sinkholes being high blood pressure, diabetes, and heart disease. In the U.S., obesity is estimated to account for 5.7% of the national health expenditure—almost (U.S.) $100 billion per year. There's also an indirect financial cost related to lost productivity due to health-related absenteeism.

The theory of premature mortality is no vague threat. Most over-fat and obese people are likely to check out before their time. Given the list of diseases noted earlier, it's not surprising that over-fat and obese people rarely reach the estimated life expectancy of 76.7 years. The social cost of premature deaths mustn't be overlooked. We have not only lost people who could have made major contributions to society, but also people who were grandmothers and grandfathers, aunts and uncles, and moms and dads to people who loved them and whom they loved, and who are now gone—thanks to excess body fat. Being over-fat doesn't automatically doom you to illness and premature death, but it certainly increases your risk of being one of the statistics.

Fat Wars is about helping to decrease the risk of premature death by moving yourself into a healthy weight range. It's about feeling better about yourself and living a different, better life. It's about understanding how the body works, and working with what nature designed. You can speed up your metabolism, burn stored body fat, increase your ability to fight disease, create more energy, increase your life expectancy, and just plain feel better. Anyone who's tried to lose fat knows it's a tough battle. The news in *Fat Wars* is that what you don't know will ensure you lose the fight. *Fat Wars* will show you how to transform your body, and make yourself the victor.

TOO SHORT FOR YOUR WEIGHT?

Is there such a thing as an ideal weight range? Yes! How do we find out what that is? Researchers who study the effects of body fat on health often refer to a person's body mass index (BMI). This is a number they calculate by using a formula that takes into account both weight and height. (Yes, size matters.) This BMI rating has become a common way to quickly judge whether your weight is putting you in a high-risk health category. For example, a study published in 1995 by Manson and colleagues followed the health of 115,000 nurses for 14 to 16 years. The lowest mortality rate was found in women with a BMI of 19 or less. The risk of premature death increased by 20% for those with BMIs in the 19 to 24.9 range, 60% for BMIs of 27 to 28.9, and doubled for those with a BMI of 29 and higher.

That same study also showed that women who kept their BMIs under 21 had no elevated risk of heart disease. When their BMIs read 21 to 25, they had a risk 30% higher, and their risk soared to 80% once their BMIs increased past 25. Researchers also found that the risks of weight-related cancers begin to rise among women whose BMI is past 26, which is quite scary, due to the fact that a BMI of 26 happens to be the average BMI of any female in North America today.

The ideal BMI is considered to be between 19 and 25. You can figure out your own BMI through a simple series of calculations that starts by dividing your weight in pounds by your height in feet squared. Then multiply this figure by 4.89. If you don't have a calculator handy, use the easy-to-follow chart below, or use the on-line calculator on *www.fatwars.com*.

How to find your body mass index (BMI): First locate your height in the left column. Then move across the chart until you hit your approximate weight. Then follow that column down to the corresponding BMI number at the bottom of the chart and *voilà*, you now know your BMI.

Fat Wars Body Mass Index Chart

Height	Body Weight in Pounds																					
4'10"	91	96	100	105	110	115	119	124	129	134	138	143	148	153	158	162	167	172	177	181	186	191
4'11"	94	99	104	109	114	119	124	128	133	138	143	148	153	158	163	168	173	178	183	188	193	198
5'0"	97	102	107	112	118	123	128	133	138	143	148	153	158	163	168	174	179	184	189	194	199	204
5'1"	100	106	111	116	122	127	132	137	143	148	153	158	164	169	174	180	185	190	195	201	206	211
5'2"	104	109	115	120	126	131	136	142	147	153	158	164	169	175	186	185	191	196	202	207	213	218
5'3"	107	113	118	124	130	135	141	146	152	158	163	169	175	180	186	191	197	203	208	214	220	225
5'4"	110	116	122	128	134	140	145	151	157	163	169	174	180	186	192	197	204	209	215	221	227	232
5'5"	114	120	126	132	138	144	150	156	162	168	174	180	186	192	198	204	210	216	222	228	234	240
5'6"	118	124	130	136	142	148	155	161	167	173	179	186	192	198	204	210	216	223	229	235	241	247
5'7"	121	127	134	140	146	153	159	166	172	178	185	191	197	204	211	217	223	230	236	242	249	255
5'8"	125	131	138	144	151	158	164	171	177	184	191	197	203	210	216	223	230	236	243	249	256	262
5'9"	128	135	142	149	155	162	169	176	182	189	196	203	209	216	223	230	236	243	250	257	263	270
5'10"	132	139	146	153	160	167	174	181	188	195	202	207	215	222	229	236	243	250	257	264	271	278
5'11"	136	143	150	157	165	172	179	186	193	200	208	215	222	229	236	243	250	257	265	272	279	286
6'0"	140	147	154	162	169	177	184	191	199	206	213	221	228	235	242	250	258	265	272	279	287	294
6'1"	144	151	159	166	174	182	189	197	204	212	219	227	235	242	250	257	265	272	280	288	295	302
6'2"	148	155	163	171	179	186	194	202	210	218	225	233	241	249	256	264	272	280	287	295	303	311
6'3"	152	160	168	176	184	192	200	208	216	224	232	240	248	256	264	272	279	287	295	303	311	319
6'4"	156	164	172	180	189	197	205	213	221	230	238	246	254	263	271	279	287	295	304	312	320	328
BMI	19	20	21	22	23	24	25	26	27	28	29	30	31	32	33	34	35	36	37	38	39	40

So What Do the Numbers Mean?

According to the National Institutes of Health, your BMI score means the following:

- under 18.5 – underweight
- 18.5–24.9 – normal
- 25–29.9 – overweight
- 30–39.9 – obese
- 40 and over – extremely obese

There is one caution with this standard, however: A lean, heavily muscled person will likely have a BMI rating that puts him or her in the danger zone, when in fact the person is healthy. Don't forget: The body is composed of lean body mass (tissue, bone, and muscle) that weighs significantly more than fat does. For example, I personally weigh 190 pounds and stand 5 feet, 8 inches tall (5.67 feet). By using the above chart or doing the calculations, I come out with a body mass index of 29.

In this particular scenario, the BMI would be wrong. (Of course it would be!) You see, I am actually in good shape. (No really, I am.) The true measure of obesity is the percentage of overall fat on the body. A normal healthy man should not exceed a body-fat percentage of 15, while the healthy limit for a woman is around 22%. I carry a body-fat percentage at the moment of 13. This is about the amount of fat a male athlete carries, and since I am an athlete of sorts, this makes sense.

A LIFE-CHANGING PLAN, NOT A DIET

You may be thinking, "Why would this Fat Wars plan be any different from all the other ones I've tried and failed at over the years?" Because *Fat Wars* is not another diet book, that's why. It is, instead, a book that is based on the science of how and why we store fat and, more importantly, the science of how to mobilize and burn the excess body fat you're now living with.

Let's face it: Most people these days would do almost anything to trim a few pounds of fat. We're desperate to fit into those old jeans that once looked oh so good on our tiny butts. We are desperate to wear a bathing suit and actually look good in it for a change. We are so desperate that, right now, one-third of all women and one-quarter of all men are on yet another diet. I say "another" diet because if the first one worked, people obviously wouldn't need the second, third, or who knows whatever number. As you will find out in the coming pages, dieting sets us up for failure time and again. Yet time and again we come back for more.

The majority of diets out there just don't work, or worse still, people can't stay on them when they do work. Most diets are unbalanced, and even though they may seem to work for a while, they usually end up creating ravenous cravings for the very foods they are deficient in. I, for one, don't like the term "diet." It conjures up negative images of short-term suffering undergone to achieve a fleeting image of beauty. Dieters soon realize that they not only gain back the fat they seemed to lose, but some extra, as a reward for their suffering.

What you need is not another short-term solution to a lifelong problem, but a lifestyle adjustment that you can work with and that works for you. In order to make a change that sticks with you *for* life, you have to make changes *in* your life. Changes that can actually fool your very genetic makeup, allowing your body to release the substance it has learned over millions of years to hold onto at all costs for survival—fat! This is, as you will soon find out, why the Fat Wars plan is and always has been so successful. *Fat Wars* is all about balance in your internal control system—your hormones. Your hormones are directly controlled by the nutrients you ingest, your environment, and your lifestyle factors (i.e., exercise).

The Fat Wars plan is designed to evoke a proper hormonal response that allows you to continuously burn fat day and night. It is a balanced approach to eating and exercise that most people find not only doable, but also enjoyable. The eating strategies you will learn allow you to see consistent results without the pain associated with dieting. As thousands of other people have learned, the Fat Wars plan is life changing.

As you begin to win your personal Fat War, you will be building muscle and losing excess fat. (Don't worry, you're not going to become a mini–Arnold Schwarzenegger just yet.) For most, this body change will not result in a high BMI rating, and the BMI will remain a useful measure. Nevertheless, it is highly advisable for anyone interested in his or her true health to get their overall fat composition measured. See the Fat Wars Web site for recommendations on how to get this done at *www.fatwars.com*.

1

The Skinny on Fat—
Why You Store It and How to Burn It

Of our 100 trillion cells, around 30 billion can store fat. These fat cells can expand to many times their natural size (in fact, up to 1,000 times). They can also shrink, but even if they shrink, they're with us for life. (The only way to make them disappear is liposuction.)

Human fat evolved over many centuries. The system worked well back in the days when the nearest mini-mart was several thousand years away. Back then, we were foraging for nuts and berries and hunting for a much-desired meal of wild game. When food was plentiful, we ate as much as we could—food storage was rarely possible in those days, and it could be some time before we had lots to eat again. Because there weren't refrigerators to store food in, we had to store the food on our bodies—as fat.

To get us through the feast/famine cycle, the human body developed the ability to convert almost anything into fat (stored fuel)—we don't have to eat fat to manufacture it. Excess dietary proteins and sugars can be turned into fat. Your body even has the ability to convert excess hormones, like insulin, into extra fat. The original plan was that this stored fuel would be used during lean times to keep us functioning.

It took thousands of years to develop this system, and it isn't going to change any time soon. In the meantime, the feast/famine cycle has been eradicated in our part of the world. Not surprisingly, this is the same part of the world that is now struggling with obesity.

The potential of your fat cells to expand is enormous, but they can also shrink. If you join the Fat Wars now, and stand up and take control of the only body you will ever own, you can change your life radically. You can be an example of what a leaner, more energetic life can bring. As you are probably aware, "fat loss" is rarely the term used when describing the transformation of one's physique and ultimately one's life. Instead, we say "weight loss," which in my strong opinion only further exacerbates an already confused topic.

The majority of our population is obsessed with their weight. You never hear someone say, "I have to lose 10 pounds of fat," but you do hear, "I have to lose 10 pounds." The question most people should be asking themselves is, "Where exactly are those 10 pounds going to come from?" Weight loss is when you are concerned with losing weight in pounds, with nary a thought as to where those pounds are coming from (i.e., lean body tissues). Fat loss, on the other hand, is what you should be interested in: the actual loss of unsightly and health-stripping body fat.

BECOMING THE MASTER OF YOUR METABOLISM

Why is it that some people can eat and eat and eat, and never seem to gain a pound, while the rest of us gain weight by just looking at food? Why is it that when a woman and a man go on the same diet (and stick to it), he seems to lose weight faster than she does? What makes the difference? The efficiency of two body processes: metabolism, which I address in this section, and thermogenesis, which I address a bit later in this chapter.

Your body is basically a living machine; it functions on millions of biochemical reactions. Every system in your body runs on the series of these reactions, which are usually fueled by the main energy system (known as the Krebs cycle). These myriad biochemical reactions require a constant supply of nutrients (i.e., vitamins, minerals, amino acids, and water) to run at peak efficiency. When the levels of various nutrients fall, the biochemical reactions fall right along with them, which means a slower metabolic rate and excess body fat. Metabolism is the series of biochemical reactions that takes place inside our systems' cells (all 100 trillion of them!) to create energy. Our bodies take the basic fuel components that we give them (carbohydrates, dietary fats, and dietary proteins, aka food) and break the fuels down to produce the energy we use to keep warm, move muscles, breathe, and blink. Our bodies either use this fuel on the spot or (you knew this was coming) store it in fat cells for later use. Of the energy that's used on the spot, approximately 80% is released as heat, while the rest does the other work. A fast, efficient metabolism can produce a lot of energy and heat (and consume a lot of fuel).

Because 80% of our energy is released as heat, we only have 20% to run our millions of biochemical reactions. Therefore, energy production (your metabolism) should never be taken for granted. To give you an idea of how a small change in energy production can affect your energy levels, all you need is a 5% reduction in this system to cause an overall energy deficit of 25%. That's called chronic fatigue syndrome.

ATP

Most people think our digestive systems break down our food and use the broken-down food directly as energy. They don't. Our bodies must first convert the carbohydrates, dietary fats, and dietary proteins into a universal energy substance. Scientists call this substance **adenosine triphosphate** (ATP). Each one of our cells has a tiny biochemical factory that can produce ATP, which is an organic compound that is stored in muscle tissue. When the brain sends a signal along the nervous system to trigger a muscle contraction, enzymes break down ATP to release the energy required for the job. In fact, we use so much ATP on a daily basis that the total amount required just to get most of us through the day would weigh in at an estimated 150 to 200 pounds. All our energy starts with ATP. It's the required basic fuel for energy that doesn't require oxygen (short-term, anaerobic efforts) and for energy that does (longer-term, aerobic efforts).

ATP is depleted rapidly. You're required to move your muscles so often (to pump your heart, scratch your head, click the remote, move a piano) that although ATP is constantly being made, it's also constantly being used up.

Going Through the Gears

ATP is the basic element of human energy, but our amazing bodies have a complex and wonderful system to keep us moving in a variety of ways. In essence, we have different gears that we can use, depending on the type of physical activity involved and how much oxygen we need at the time. Think of it as shifting the gears in a car.

First Gear: ATP

For immediate energy, we can get along just by using ATP. Our bodies make this constantly, but it's not stored as pure ATP in large quantities. ATP alone can power our muscles when we throw a ball or swing a tennis racquet—efforts that last for less than three seconds.

Second Gear: ATP, CP

For a more sustained effort, the muscles pull in a second fuel component, **creatine phosphate (CP).** This is an energy source that can be stored longer than ATP and is available to juice up the fuel mix when ATP runs out. What's really happening is that CP donates its phosphate atom to what's left after ATP is broken down. *Voilà*, we have enough ATP to keep us going for up to 10 seconds. During this time, we can do a sprint or wrestle a pair of shoes onto a small child.

Third Gear: ATP, CP, Glucose . . . and Lactic Acid

If we need energy for more than 10 seconds—say, for up to two minutes—we go into third gear. At this point, the muscles are using ATP and calling on CP to help make more quick fuel. In addition, glucose and glycogen (stored sugars) are being broken down to help turn more spent ATP into usable fuel. A by-product of the glucose breakdown is lactic acid. Hydrogen ions released from excess lactic acid make our muscles burn—a clear signal to our bodies to either stop what they're doing because they don't have the fuel to go any further or add oxygen to the fuel mix. Time to take a deep breath and go to the next level.

Fourth Gear: Oxygen Overdrive (the Aerobic Phase)

If your body's energy needs are for longer than two minutes, you must add oxygen to the fuel mix in order to carry on. Let's face it—most of the things we do last longer than two minutes. This is where conditioning comes in: Oxygen utilization is a key indicator of fitness. That's because the more efficiently our bodies can use oxygen, the longer we're able to generate enough energy for long-term, strenuous effort (and the more fat we burn).

At this stage, we're still making ATP, but another part of the muscle cell (the mitochondria) kicks in to produce long-term energy. It combines a number of elements, including oxygen and fatty acids (YES!), which burn nicely to produce a sustained source of energy for activity. This is the gear that burns fat.

Don't worry if you're not sure how to get your body into fourth gear; I go into that in Chapters 13 and 14.

Boosting Your Metabolism to Burn Fat

Because muscle is a prime site for fat burning, one way to get the fat burners working better is by moving those muscles through proper exercise (I'll cover exercise in Chapter 13). In addition, a higher-protein diet has been proven to increase thermogenic activity (more on this in Chapter 8). A 1993 study by Dr. Barenys and his colleagues at Rovira University in Spain found that the combination of a higher-protein diet and moderate exercise increases the body's metabolic activity much more than a high-protein diet alone or exercise alone. The combination of a higher-protein diet and exercise was so effective that it raised the resting metabolic rate of the participants well into the day following the exercise.

According to research by Dr. Donald Layman of the University of Illinois Medical School in Urbana-Champaign, higher-protein diets help people maintain muscle mass during weight loss, which is important for controlling metabolic rate. The reason for this metabolic enhancement may lie in dietary protein's ability to increase your metabolism by enhancing the action of the thyroid gland. A protein meal can increase your metabolic rate by 25% to 30%, compared with an increase of 4% after a high-carbohydrate meal.

UNDERSTANDING THERMOGENESIS: THE KEY TO BURNING EXCESS BODY FAT

Thermogenesis is a subordinate to metabolism. Think of it this way: Metabolism is the generator of our systems, creating energy from the fuels that we consume so that the body can carry out its trillions of tasks every day. Thermogenesis is like a furnace that creates extra heat for the body by burning excess calories from our fat supplies.

Metabolism provides both heat and energy so that we can go about our daily tasks; thermogenesis just provides heat. Why do we have this auxiliary system? We are warm-blooded creatures who have to keep our body temperatures at a constant level—98.6°F (37°C)—in a changing environment. Our bodies work hard to regulate our own temperature. This is a very big job, and we always need to produce heat.

> ### How Heat Is Made
> In general, heat is produced in three ways:
> - through physical activity, during which the muscles create heat as they do work, enabling them to do double duty efficiently (metabolism);
> - through diet-induced activity, especially when you've had a large meal that requires your digestive system to go into overdrive (metabolism). (Do you ever notice how hot it gets after a holiday dinner?);
> - through temperature regulation, when your skeletal muscle cells "shiver" to warm up your body (shivering thermogenesis).

In thermogenesis, stored energy (body fat) is burned to produce heat. The chemical production of heat within the body promotes the oxidation of body fat. In order for your body to maintain a temperature of 98.6°F (37°C), it must constantly burn fat. The efficiency of your thermogenic systems can mean the difference between average or overabundant fat stores.

As shown in Figure 1-1, there are actually two types of fat cells in your body:

- White fat cells, referred to as white adipose tissue (WAT). The excess body fat that you have learned to hate is composed of WAT cells. WAT cells are mostly inert due to their extremely low levels of mitochondria (which are sort of like molecular motors). WAT cells are ideal storage containers for future energy needs.
- Brown fat cells, referred to as brown adipose tissue (BAT). BAT cells are loaded with mitochondria, which is how they earned their name in the first place—mitochondria have a brownish hue. The function of the BAT cells is to provide extra heat by burning body fat or to create thermogenesis. BAT cells also burn the calories your body doesn't need. Fat buildup can occur when the BAT cells are not working properly or not being activated often enough.

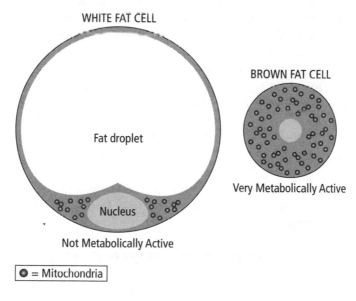

Figure 1-1: *White and brown fat cells.*

More on the Good Fat: BAT

Now before you get too excited about your new discovery that some fat cells in your body may actually be allies, I have to stifle some of your enthusiasm and inform you that we humans have an extremely low quantity of BAT cells. But don't despair, because science has hinted at ways in which you can increase the number and activity of these little fat burners, as I discuss later.

You are well aware of those individuals who seem to be able to eat anything they want without gaining weight (it's surprising these people have any friends). These are the same people who have been asked over and over again, "Where does it all go?" The answer may be that these fortunate people are walking around with an excess of BAT cells, or that their BAT cells are a lot more productive than yours or mine.

It's theorized that the sudden weight gain experienced by many between the ages of 30 and 40 may be the result of a shutdown of the BAT cell/thermogenic mechanism, under the influence of some genetic cue. When that shutdown happens, we must find ways to reactivate BAT cell thermogenesis and reverse the genetic trigger. Otherwise, we will continue to store body fat, no matter what we try.

The process of waking up your slumbering BAT cells starts with mobilizing stored body fat (through proper exercise, dietary hormonal control, and nutrient intervention) and transporting it effectively to the BAT cells (and muscle cells) where it is incinerated, i.e., eradicated through thermogenesis. Over time, an active thermogenic system may be able to generate the production of additional BAT cells, resulting in a dramatic increase in the amount of fat that you burn as fuel.

Research has shown that BAT cells can be increased in humans who are exposed to cold temperatures for long periods of time (such as people living in the Arctic). If moving to the Arctic seems too drastic a step to take in order to burn fat, science has also isolated an ally from Mother Nature called *Citrus aurantium* (or Bitter Orange or *zhi shi*), which is a South Asian fruit that resembles a small orange. It contains five key phytochemicals called alkaloids that increase the breakdown of stored fat and enhance the metabolic rate through thermogenesis. It shows great promise in stimulating the fat-burning process (more on this important nutrient in Chapter 12).

Warming up the Engine: More Ways to Create Heat

Thermogenesis helps keep you warm even when you don't require muscular energy. As explained earlier, unlike metabolism that creates energy for the body, thermogenesis just burns extra fat to create heat. Thermogenesis is what keeps animals warm during hibernation and newborn babies warm before their metabolic systems have developed. It keeps you and me warm when we're sleeping. But you can also think of thermogenesis as your personal metabolic helper.

Your personal heating system uses three specialized chemical proteins, called uncoupling proteins (UCPs), that convert food energy into heat instead of ATP. Our sources of these three chemical proteins are BAT, muscle tissue, immune cells, white adipose tissue (WAT), and skeletal muscles; the proteins are found throughout the body. These chemical proteins are called uncoupling proteins to distinguish them from the proteins that are used when generating energy to create both heat and energy; uncoupling proteins, on the other hand, can separate the work of producing heat from energy production and make only heat. If this sounds too complicated, don't worry, all you have to realize is that these UCPs are big-time allies in the Fat Wars.

Thermogenesis relies on the most abundant and economical source of fuel it can find to produce the heat: your body fat. You need the body fat that you are at war with to help keep your temperature running at 98.6°F (37°C) in the shade. This is why you always need *some* body fat in storage. The problem is that the majority of us have enough fuel stored away to heat a medium-sized crowd in addition to ourselves (and we keep thinking we have a fuel shortage).

The heating process starts by mobilizing fat from the fat cells and carrying the fat through the blood into the muscle cells. In the muscle cells, UCPs convert the fat to soluble fat so that it can be incinerated. As the body becomes more efficient at moving the fat through the system (that is, as BAT cells and UCPs, in particular, start working effectively), you get slimmer and slimmer. The Fat Wars plan is designed to help stimulate both your metabolic and thermogenic systems by balancing the necessary hormones that regulate this process.

CONNECTING THE THYROID WITH METABOLISM AND THERMOGENESIS

The thyroid is a major player in both the thermogenic and metabolic processes. This gland, located at the front of the neck, produces different endocrine hormones (hormones that travel through the bloodstream to distant targets) that regulate both processes.

Numerous North Americans suffer from a sluggish thyroid, the technical name for which is hypothyroidism. And since the thyroid gland is the thermostat that controls the regulation station of our metabolism, many overweight North Americans may be suffering from a slow metabolism due to a sluggish thyroid. How many North Americans, you ask? Enough to fill over 36 million thyroid prescriptions a year.

Three Little Hormones

Three separate hormones are produced by the thyroid gland. The primary thyroid hormone is called T4 (thyroxine); it's not very active. T4 is converted within the peripheral tissue to T3 (triiodothyronine), which is the most active of the thyroid hormones (it's up to eight times more active than T4). The conversion of T4 to T3 is dependent on the enzyme 5-deiodinase, which cannot be formed without the mineral selenium. Millions of North Americans consume only limited quantities of selenium, because of soil depletion and overprocessing of food, among other things.

The thyroid gland also produces a relatively inactive hormone called reverse T3 (rT3). In fact, almost 40% of your T4 is converted into this inactive form. Obviously, T3 is where the majority of the action is, especially where your fat-loss goals are concerned.

This, by no means, is a reason to blame all of your fat woes on your thyroid gland. Millions of people have normal functioning thyroid glands, yet still suffer from excess body fat. Even those people who do have a sluggish thyroid can stay relatively trim through following the Fat Wars eating and exercise strategy. For an in-depth understanding of how the thyroid gland works, please see *www.fatwars.com* (thyroid icon).

Testing for a Sluggish Thyroid

The most common indicators of hypothyroidism include: cold hands and feet, high cholesterol, high blood pressure, depression, constant fatigue, sleepiness, muscle weakness, brittle fingernails and hair, dry skin, chronic constipation, and weight gain.

A couple of years ago, I had the opportunity to interview one of the leading thyroid specialists in the U.S. on my daily radio show *Body Talk*. Dr. Ridha Arem, associate professor of medicine in the Division of Endocrinology and Metabolism at Baylor College of Medicine in Houston, Texas, indicated that weight gain should be a reason for thyroid testing, particularly if you are also suffering from emotional and physical symptoms of hypothyroidism.

Caution: If you are diagnosed with hypothyroidism, there are certain foods that should not be consumed in excess. These foods contain goitrogens, substances that enlarge the thyroid. Goitrogen-rich foods have been shown to inhibit the enzymatic reactions that convert T4 into the metabolically active T3. These foods are: soybeans, broccoli, Brussels sprouts, cabbage, cauliflower, kale, watercress, mustard greens, rutabaga, spinach, turnips, peaches, and pears. Don't get me wrong, these foods have a lot of nutritional value. But in the case of hypothyroid disorder, I do not recommend consuming them in any great quantities. Please check with your health professional first.

If you suspect that you may be one of the thousands of North Americans with a less-than-superb metabolism that's the result of a sluggish thyroid gland, a qualified health professional can help you in many ways. In order to personally (as opposed to professionally) assess the functionality of your thyroid, you can perform a simple procedure in your own home called the thyroid temperature test (TTT). The TTT is advocated by many physicians and can easily be followed up by various tests that clinically assess the need for hormonal therapy. For instructions on how to perform the TTT, please refer to the Fat Wars Web site at *www.fatwars.com*.

Leptin—the Newest Weapon in the Fat Wars

Leptin is a hormone produced by fat cells (as well as endothelial cells and immune cells). Leptin acts on nerve cells in the brain (and elsewhere), to regulate body weight by decreasing food intake and increasing energy expenditure (the burning of excess fat). Leptin may well be one of the most important biochemical messengers in controlling our metabolism. The more active your leptin, the higher your metabolic rate.

Most of the interest in leptin as a possible anti-obesity agent started in 1995, due to research conducted by Dr. Jeffrey Friedman and colleagues in New York. Dr. Friedman's group discovered that mice that were lacking the gene for leptin became obese. When the researchers injected leptin into these mice, their fat stores began to shrink considerably. The researchers concluded that under normal conditions, fat cells secrete leptin to inform the brain how fat the body is, and therefore whether an organism should keep eating or stop eating. We are all born with approximately 30 billion of the little fat tanks, and they're not going anywhere. Dieting only shrinks fat cells. Although shrunken, they readily expand again, which is why it's so hard for ex-dieters to stay slim.

But new research may change all that. In 1997, a team of researchers at the University of Georgia discovered that leptin actually causes the death of fat cells rather than simply reducing them in size. This process, referred to as apoptosis, explains why rats injected with leptin remain thin long after treatment.

A six-month study presented in June 1998 at an American Diabetes Association conference by Amgen Inc., a clinical research facility in California, reported that eight moderately obese people who were given the highest dose of leptin lost an average of 16 pounds, while 37 others who took lower doses lost much less weight (as little as 1.5 pounds).

When you skip meals, as so many people do these days, leptin levels decline, leading to changes in thyroid hormones that ultimately slow your metabolic rate. The result is that you have a much harder time losing fat. In obese individuals, leptin does not work properly. Obese individuals tend to produce an excessive amount of the hormone, but it's as if the body becomes unreceptive to the hormonal message (almost like insulin resistance in Type 2 diabetes). Even if your thyroid hormones are being produced in sufficient quantities, if the message of leptin is not being heard then the thyroid hormones will be less effective at increasing your metabolism. On the other hand, if there is not enough of the potent T3 thyroid hormone being produced, leptin will be powerless to enhance your metabolism.

A new study presented last year in the journal *Life Science* showed that obese individuals tend to have very low levels of the mineral zinc (referred to as hypozincemia), and that zinc treatment was able to increase leptin production by a whopping 142%. The data from this study suggest that zinc may play an important role in the mediation of leptin production.

Obesity researchers are presently conducting ongoing human trials with leptin in hopes of finding new ways to control body-fat levels. The study of leptin is still in its infancy, but the potential leptin holds for the treatment of obesity is enormous (see *www.fatwars.com* for regular updates on leptin research).

EXPRESS YOURSELF

As you are now well aware, the potential of your fat cells to expand is enormous. But the same potential also exists for shrinkage. If you constantly exceed your body's needs by eating too much and exercising too little, or the wrong way (see Chapter 13), then you will no doubt join the millions of other over-fat people around the globe who are already sorry for their choices. But if you join the Fat Wars now, and stand up and take control of the only body you will ever own, you can reap the benefits of more energy, more optimism, and much better health.

Throughout *Fat Wars*, you will learn that the factors that control your genetic makeup, the switches, in a sense, that make you gain or lose fat, are not fixed entities. They are well within your control. You can't tinker with your genes. But the way those genes are expressed, which is referred to as your phenotype, is up to you. After all, you can't blame your genes for the last time you pigged out on a double cheeseburger, French fries, and of course we can't forget the diet Coke.

KEY TACTICS

1. Each and every one of us has around 30 billion fat cells that can expand to many times their natural size (in fact, up to 1,000 times).
2. With the guidelines presented in *Fat Wars*, these fat cells can also greatly shrink. It is a reduction in body fat, not overall weight, that is the key to health.
3. Fat loss is controlled by our metabolism. As we learn to change our metabolism, we learn how to control fat loss.

2

Fat Burning—

The Hormonal Connection

Tammy is an incredible lady. She has a full-time career as a radio producer and a part-time career as a professional announcer and radio host. She is fun loving and dedicated to her daily workout. In fact, Tammy never misses her evening boxersize classes for fear of gaining extra weight. She's tried almost every diet ever invented, and even thought up a couple of her own. All failed miserably.

About one year ago, Tammy came to see me about her frustrations with never-ending diets and her continual increase in weight. After carefully reviewing the foods she ate and her exercise routine and taking a fat-percentage measurement, I recognized that Tammy was eating too many processed carbohydrates and not getting enough dietary proteins. Tammy was also doing "too much" of the wrong kind of exercise. I realized that Tammy probably couldn't lose her extra fat because she had a high resting insulin level and an elevated stress response. This condition was not only stopping her body from burning fat as a fuel source, but was also dampening her metabolism. Unfortunately, millions of over-fat people around the world have the same problem as Tammy.

I suggested that she reduce her consumption of processed carbohydrates and replace the processed carbs with unrefined carbohydrates (such as whole grains, vegetables, and fruit). I also recommended increasing her dietary proteins and adding some essential fats, especially the omega-3s, to her dismal diet. I encouraged Tammy to eat more frequently (five to six times a day) and to supplement two of her meals with high-protein shakes. If that wasn't enough, I also suggested that Tammy cut down on her aerobic exercise and start resistance training (using weights) two or three times a week.

Needless to say, none of these suggestions made any sense to Tammy. "Carbohydrates don't make me fat! How could they? They don't contain any fat to begin with!" And "You want me to eat five or six meals a day! How do you think I got fat in the first place?" And worst of all, "You want me to cut down on my fat-burning exercise and bulk up with weights?!" Did Tammy follow my advice? Not a chance! It went counter to everything she had ever heard about losing weight.

Now fast-forward almost one year. My phone rings. "Brad, it's Tammy. Guess what?" The pitch of her voice was rising in excitement. "I've lost nearly 20 pounds, and it's all due to your advice!" Tammy proceeded to tell me that she had literally come to her wits' end almost two months earlier. "If I'd gained just one more pound on another crummy diet and exercise plan, I would have killed myself," she said.

In desperation, Tammy remembered the consultation from months earlier. Figuring she had failed at every other weight-loss approach, she decided to give my recommendations a go. In just a few days, after lowering her refined carbs, eating smaller meals more frequently, and switching to the exercise routine I designed for her, Tammy could hardly believe how the fat started melting off. Twenty pounds of energy-sapping fat had soon packed up and left the premises. The amazing thing is that Tammy is just one example of thousands who have benefited from the recommendations set forth in Fat Wars.

Millions of frustrated and confused men and women have the same out-dated beliefs that kept Tammy from losing weight. They cling to these beliefs, even though research and years of continual weight-loss failure have shown that they need to be replaced. Worse, many men and women sit still and do nothing, hoping that one day their excess lard will magically vanish when some magic fat-loss pill is finally invented. Unfortunately, you probably won't live to see such a pill in your lifetime.

OUR GENES, OUR GREAT-GRANDPARENTS' GENES, OUR GREAT-GREAT-GREAT . . .

We've all heard the saying, "You are what you eat." Well, when it comes to how our fat cells behave, we also are what our ancestors ate. According to Dr. Boyd Eaton, an expert in evolution and the diet of early humans, 99% of our genetic structure was formed before our biological ancestors evolved into Homo sapiens, about 40,000 years ago. And 99.99% of our genes were formed before the advent of agriculture, about 10,000 years ago.

> ### Feast and Famine
> You're able to read this book right now because your ancestors had the necessary machinery (physiological and biochemical) to convert any excess calories they consumed into fat that they used to weather future famines. You are no different in this regard. So even though you may know (all too well) that you are going to be eating again soon, your body doesn't. Kind of like socks for Christmas— you may not want them, but you get them anyway, this trait (your physiological and biochemical machinery, that is) is a gift from your prehistoric ancestors to you.

Our need for specific nutrients is embedded in our genes and has evolved through millions of years. In fact, our genes—which control every function in our bodies—are essentially the same as those of our early ancestors. If we give our bodies what our genes have programmed them for, our genes will do their job well and we will stay healthy. But if we give our bodies unfamiliar substances or nutrients in the wrong ratios, our bodies will eventually malfunction, which leads to disease. A sober example of this is found in the way prescription drugs interact with our biochemical makeup. Even though these drugs are designed to help the patient in one area or another, they all contain molecules that did not exist in our bodies as we were evolving. Consequently these same prescription medications cause many side effects along with their specific benefits. If there is a man-made chemical of one sort or another in something we eat, the same principle applies. These chemicals cannot fit exactly into our biochemical locks, so they could be interfering with the right keys for unlocking health. Science has developed more than 100,000 chemicals that were never part of our evolution. It's kind of like having an incredible vehicle that is designed to take you anywhere you want to go—in style—but carelessly placing the wrong fuels in the tank until the vehicle eventually breaks down and ends up in the scrapyard. Even though this is a crude metaphor, your vehicle (i.e., your body) isn't replaceable, which is something I believe too many of us never even think about.

So what are we supposed to eat then? What did our ancestors eat? A diet far different from what we're eating today. We are consumers of a modern diet, rich in refined carbohydrates and over-processed dietary fats. Genetically, we are prepared for a diet of wild game and unprocessed fruits, vegetables, nuts, and seeds. But things have changed in the last 100 centuries.

Today, we have lost touch with the fundamental principles that shaped our physiology and gotten away from the capabilities of the genes that got us this far in the first place. Instead of eating like our ancestors, we have become carbohydrate addicts. We are consuming carbohydrates as our main source of food, with dietary proteins as the supplement. Dr. Eaton also has concluded, through extensive research, that the early human diet consisted of at least 30% protein. In 1985, statistics from the National Research Council in America reported that the average American diet consisted of 46% carbohydrates, 43% fats (and not the good ones), and only 11% protein.

So what does this have to do with obesity? A lot!

According to geneticists, it takes between 1,000 and 10,000 generations for any substantial genetic alterations to become part of our destiny. Since we've been consuming carbohydrates as our main food source for only 10,000 years (and highly processed carbohydrates for less than 100 years), it may take another 10,000 years for our genes to catch up with this high-carbohydrate diet. Dr. Eaton believes that the less we eat like our ancestors, the more susceptible we become to many of the diseases of modern civilization, such as diabetes, heart disease, arthritis, cancer, and let's not forget, obesity.

In order to win the Fat Wars and become healthy, we must eat what our bodies are genetically receptive to. Since our hunter-gatherer brothers and sisters from centuries ago functioned best on a diet rich in proteins from lean meat, supplemented with whole fruits, vegetables, nuts, and seeds, we would be wise to do the same. The forces of natural selection allowed us to evolve to function optimally on these foods. And since food was not always in abundance, and we didn't have the convenience or guarantee of at least three balanced meals per day, we developed an incredible storage capacity within our 30 billion fat cells. Don't forget: Each and every one of those 30 billion fat cells can expand 1,000 times in volume, and if that isn't enough, they can also increase in number (yikes!).

The French Paradox

The French enjoy just as much meat and fish as we do, but they also consume nearly four times as much butter and twice as much cheese (all fat-laden foods) as us. If we ate that way, our doctors and nutritionists would probably warn that it will eventually kill us! So why don't our friends on the Mediterranean suffer from these diseases to the same extent that we do? The answer may lie in the fact that they consume only about 18% as much sugar as North Americans do.

YOUR HORMONES—THE THREE HEAVY HITTERS

As I have mentioned, we are all born with a unique series of genetic information—a blueprint of sorts—called our genotype. Our genotype has been handed down through many generations, and it sets many of us up for the continual storage of body fat for survival. As in the vehicle analogy I used earlier, your genes do not necessarily dictate the outcome of events, but instead are strongly influenced by the types of fuel you choose to consume. These fuels, along with proper exercise and rest, stimulate your hormonal system to send either positive (fat-burning) or negative (fat-storing) messages to your body's cells.

These hormones dictate how your "machine" is going to run. The interaction of your genotype with your total environment is known as your phenotype. It's your phenotype that matters, and it's your phenotype that is under your control. Nature may have given you the physical equivalent of a Volvo or a Maserati, but you decide whether to run it on cheap or premium fuel, whether to drive it in the desert without a break, and whether to ignore the need for a tune up.

Hormone One: Insulin, a Double Agent

The body has many hormones at work—nearly 30 that we know of, with many more to be found—but only a few are involved in fat gain and loss. Insulin, a polypeptide hormone that is secreted from the beta cells of the pancreas in an area called the islets of Langerhans, is one of them. Insulin is secreted immediately following a meal and during periods of elevated blood sugar. Your diet directly affects insulin production.

Insulin is the Dr. Jekyll and Mr. Hyde of metabolism. On the positive side, insulin performs functions necessary for life, including the deposit of sugar (glycogen) and amino acids (protein) in muscle and the synthesis of chemical proteins for building enzymes, hormones, and muscle. On the negative side, when insulin is produced in excess, it plays a major role in obesity by increasing the synthesis (manufacture) of body fat while inhibiting the breakdown of stored body fat for use as a fuel. Insulin is also a major contributor to the number one killer in North America, cardiovascular disease, as well as to Type 2 diabetes.

Insulin and Diabetes

When most of us think of insulin, we tend to think of diabetes. There are several types of diabetes, but you are probably most familiar with the two most common types. Type 1, which is also referred to as juvenile diabetes, accounts for 10% of the disorders known as diabetes. Type 1 diabetes is due to a dysfunction of the pancreas, which is unable to secrete either any insulin or enough to lower blood-glucose levels.

Type 2 diabetes is a whole different problem, accounting for almost 90% of diabetes disorders. Type 2 diabetes, or adult-onset diabetes, is caused when the insulin receptor sites in the cells become insensitive to the hormone. When insulin cannot bind to the cells to allow the sugar to enter them, blood sugar can't leave the bloodstream. Instead, both blood-sugar and blood insulin levels remain elevated. (Impaired glucose tolerance is a precondition of diabetes and affects many more people than does diabetes. Again, the muscle and liver cells that store the blood sugar as glycogen don't work well with insulin. The transport proteins inside the cells that help bring in the sugar are working at a slow pace, and more insulin is needed to push the sugar into the cells.)

Over time, elevated blood-sugar levels, along with high insulin levels, can lead to a whole array of physiological changes, which are collectively referred to as Syndrome X. The term "Syndrome X" was first coined in 1988 by Dr. Gerald Reaven, an endocrinologist from Stanford University. Dr. Reaven defined it as a clustering of interrelated symptoms that always includes insulin resistance. Syndrome X is believed to be caused by eating too many processed high-carbohydrate foods, such as white-flour-based products, corn products, and junk food. Over-fat and obese people tend to suffer a lot more from hyperinsulinemia (high blood insulin) than their thinner counterparts.

Insulin and Fat Storage

Because insulin is especially sensitive to dietary carbohydrates—they are metabolized into sugar—the more carbohydrates you eat at one time, the greater the amount of insulin needed to clear the sugar from the bloodstream. Refined carbs, such as white flour, pasta, bread, cookies, chips, etc., are especially good at raising your insulin levels. Once you realize that at any time of the day or night, your entire bloodstream (if you are non-diabetic) only contains approximately 5 grams (about 1 teaspoon) of glucose (blood sugar), you may appreciate how easy it is to disrupt this delicate balance. So the next time you reach for something like a cinnamon bun, realize that the 12 teaspoons of sugar (not including the white flour) that are released into your body will most definitely cause hormonal mayhem. You will recognize the feeling as a temporary burst of energy, quickly followed by a need to curl into a ball and hibernate.

And if that's not enough to scare you, here's the real kicker—insulin is the major biochemical messenger of fat storage. Your body is naturally designed to draw upon fat (instead of sugar) for 70% of its energy needs during day-to-day activities (not including exercise). But high insulin levels prevent your body from using fat for fuel and instead seek alternative sources, such as glucose and amino acids.

Insulin controls our rate of fat storage (lipogenesis) by first stimulating transporters in the fat cells to take up fat and sugar from the bloodstream. Insulin then calls upon a lipogenic (fat storing) enzyme, lipoprotein lipase (LPL), that's responsible for setting up the necessary biochemical reactions within the cell that eventually stores the fat and sugar as body fat (see Figure 2-1), and worse yet, making sure it stays there. Insulin also lowers the amount of a special transporter protein, carnitine, that is responsible for shuttling longer-chain fatty acids into the mitochondria of our cells to be burned as fuel. Without sufficient quantities of carnitine to transport these larger fats into our metabolic engines, fat burning quickly comes to a halt.

Insulin likes to invest in prime fat-cell property as we get older. It starts to concentrate the majority of its fat-storing investments in the middle of the body, within the abdomen and around the vital organs. On the one hand, this is the worst place to have excess fat, because of increased health risks. On the other hand, belly fat is one of the easiest fats to get rid of. This may be due to its higher metabolic activity than subcutaneous fat (under the skin), such as fat on the hips and thighs.

Forty-six percent of the calories in the typical North American diet are composed of carbohydrates (primarily processed carbs). Those carbohydrates must be broken down into sugars, and either used as immediate energy, stored as short-term energy (as glycogen), or turned into fat. But those sugars cannot get into your fat cells and take up residence without our old friend insulin.

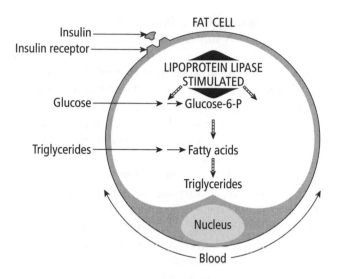

Figure 2-1: *Too much insulin boosts fat storage by activating lipoprotein lipase.*

You only have a limited capacity to store short-term carbohydrate energy (glycogen); even obese people can only store 1 to 2 pounds of carbohydrates as glycogen. This is why the remainder of any excess sugars (carbohydrates) from your diet eventually find their way into our fat cells and we get fatter and fatter. According to Sam Graci, nutritional researcher and author of *The Food Connection*, here's what normally happens when you eat a typical refined-carbohydrate meal and insulin is stimulated:

- 30% of the sugar, as glucose, is used to form immediate energy while your fat lays idle;
- 30% is stored as short-term energy (glycogen) in your liver (where the brain accesses its fuel) and in your muscles;
- 40% of the sugar is stored as long-term energy (body fat).

What I haven't told you up until now is that most individuals consume approximately 3 pounds of sugar per week (156 pounds per year). And because we only have a limited capacity to store short-term carbohydrate energy, our glycogen tanks are always full. If our liver and muscle glycogen reserves are never being depleted because we are constantly consuming sugars, then insulin must find another way to deal with the excess sugar. There's really no place left to store it other than in the fat cells. So now here's what happens when you eat your next high-carbohydrate meal:

- 30% of the sugar is used as immediate energy;
- 70% of the sugar is stored as body fat.

In other words, when you keep insulin levels high by constantly con-suming large quantities of processed carbohydrates, your body has no choice but to store the sugar in your 30 billion fat cells since your glycogen tanks are full. Excess insulin not only makes you fat, it keeps you fat! In order to free up the fat so that it can be burned in the muscle cells, you've got to lower your insulin levels.

So just how do we lower our insulin levels? By changing our diet and exercising properly. We can also try supplementing our diet by taking cer-tain nutrients that increase insulin sensitivity (see Chapter 12).

Many scientists, physicians, and weight-loss experts believe the key to successful long-term fat loss is in balancing our insulin levels, lower-ing our glucose load, and increasing our protein intake. By now you likely understand that avoiding sugar isn't the whole answer. The fact is, virtually every carbohydrate you consume (bagels, potatoes, carrots, and breads, for example) is eventually, and most times too quickly, meta-bolized into glucose (sugar) in your system. You'll find out just how quickly in Part II. The higher your glucose load, the higher your insulin levels. Understanding how insulin levels relate to increased fat gain will give you the knowledge to keep your 30 billion fat cells from growing exponentially.

HORMONE TWO: GLUCAGON

Glucagon acts as the antagonist hormone to insulin. Glucagon and insulin are the two master controllers of your metabolism. Glucagon, like insulin, is a polypeptide hormone that is secreted from the pancreas, but from the alpha cells. Insulin is responsible for controlling blood sugar by clearing it from the bloodstream before it gets too high; glucagon is respon-sible for preventing the blood sugar from falling too low, which can hap-pen when you skip meals, overexercise, or restrict your calories too severely (as on many diets).

As you are now well aware, carbohydrates have a very powerful stim-ulatory effect on insulin, whereas certain amino acids (from protein) only have a slight effect. On the other hand, being an opposing hormone to insulin, glucagon is greatly stimulated by protein intake, while sugars act as a potent glucagon inhibitor. In a very real sense, what is good for insulin is not so good for glucagon.

Just as insulin sets the stage for fat gain, glucagon sets the stage for fat loss (see Figure 2-2). The problem is, when equivalent levels of both hormones are present, insulin always prevails. The hormones exert opposing actions on the two key enzymes that control the fate of fat in your body; the first hormone you have already been introduced to, LPL (controlled by insulin), but the one you really want to get familiar with is its subordinate, hormone-sensitive lipase (HSL).

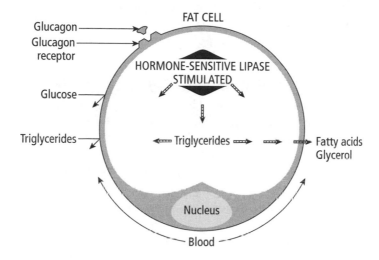

Figure 2-2: *Glucagon stimulates hormone-sensitive lipase, which encourages fat burning.*

HSL performs the opposite functions of LPL by causing the release of fat from fat cells. Once released, the fat can be shipped to other cells and burned as fuel. The important thing to note is that HSL activity increases as glucagon is stimulated (through controlled carbohydrate and protein intake), while LPL activity increases when insulin is high, especially after a meal that's high in carbs and low in protein.

It's Up to You

Make no mistake about it: This metabolic tug of war that takes place every time you eat is directly under your control. You have the ability to alter your metabolism toward fat burning instead of fat storing by changing how you eat (I explain this in Part III). By choosing the right foods, you can determine which process will prevail. So instead of allowing your metabolism to control you, you can control it. If you choose to flood your body with insulin, then expect your fat cells to inflate by becoming fat-storing machines. But if you choose to have a proper hormonal balance between glucagon and insulin, then expect your fat cells to deflate while your body becomes a fat-burning machine.

> **A Recap**
> High insulin levels stimulate the release and action of the fat-storing enzyme, lipoprotein lipase, ultimately making you fatter while inhibiting fat from being released from your fat cells. Glucagon stimulates the release and action of the fat-releasing, hormone-sensitive enzyme lipase, which mobilizes fat for energy, causing you to lose body fat.

HORMONE THREE: HUMAN GROWTH HORMONE

Human growth hormone (HGH) is a protein-based hormone released by the anterior pituitary gland in the center of your brain. One of its main jobs is to regulate growth, especially at puberty, but its role goes much beyond that. HGH is also responsible for increasing lean body mass (muscle) and decreasing stored body fat, by freeing it up as an energy source.

HGH is secreted in rhythms throughout the day and night, but it's primarily secreted while we sleep. In fact, up to 75% of HGH is produced while we are in our deepest phase of sleep (Stages III and IV). It is also produced in response to intense exercise (especially resistance training). The pulsing effect of HGH is regulated by two opposing hormones produced in the hypothalamus, a gland that sits just above the pituitary. One of these hormones (growth hormone–releasing hormone [GHRH]) is responsible for increasing the amount of HGH in the bloodstream; the second hormone (somatostatin) is responsible for decreasing or halting the production of HGH.

The circadian pattern of HGH secretion is roughly as follows:
- 7 a.m. — low
- 9 a.m. — medium
- 11 a.m. — low
- noon — high
- 2 to 5 p.m. — low and medium peaks
- 7 p.m. — medium/high
- midnight — large bursts (if asleep by 9 p.m.)
- 3 to 6 a.m. — small peaks

Three factors are important in achieving optimal natural secretions:
- going to bed early, with sound sleep from 11 p.m. to 2 a.m.;
- having regular, strenuous exercise;
- remaining free of disease.

HGH only hangs around for a few minutes after it's pumped into our bloodstream. Although its appearance is fleeting, it is very powerful. In those few minutes, HGH has a mission—it must make its way to two locations. One is fat cells, where it latches onto specific growth hormone receptors, activating the release of stored fat for energy. The other location is the liver, where it stimulates the release of a special set of hormones called insulin-like growth factors (IGF), sometimes called somatomedins. These growth factors bear a close resemblance in structure to insulin, thus their names. The various IGFs are required for the growth of the cells, bones, muscles, organs, and the immune system. Even though HGH stimulates the release of these growth factors, they are also created independently.

HGH on the Decline

After our early 20s, HGH declines approximately 14% per decade; around the age of 60 we have experienced an 80% decline in the hormone. IGF levels follow closely behind, with a decline of nearly 50% soon after middle age (40). It is widely believed that these prodigious declines of HGH and IGF are directly responsible for robbing us of our youth, and for the body transformations that we have all come to fear. The loss of lean body mass as we age is a biological trait shared by the majority of the population; it reflects the downward spiral of HGH.

Nature's Way to Higher HGH Levels

Nearly 50% of the pituitary gland, where HGH is produced, is composed of growth hormone–producing cells (called somatotrophes). The amazing thing is that these cells can be stimulated to produce youthful amounts of HGH at any age. In 1995, Dr. William Sonntag and his colleagues at the Bowman Gray School of Medicine in North Carolina completed a study showing that the age-related decline in HGH secretion is actually reversible. The best approach for increasing growth hormone and its growth-factor family is to supply the body with ways to increase its supply naturally. That way the body won't build up a defense mechanism that can eventually cut off the supply of this essential hormone.

Bioavailable IGF and its growth-factor friends are naturally occurring in exceptionally high concentrations in life's first food, colostrum—that first secretion of mother's milk after birth. Antiaging clinics around the world have isolated growth hormone and its growth-factor family, charging exorbitant fees for something found naturally and in perfect balance in colostrum. The added benefit of colostrum is that these muscle-building, fat-burning growth factors are not degraded by our systems. Instead, they enter our bloodstreams intact. Even better news is that bovine colostrum can be found on your local health-food store shelves. Given the fact that two-thirds of our population will lose one-third of their muscle by the time they are 60, we can use all the natural help we can get!

Human-Growth-Hormone Injections

Many studies have demonstrated both physical and mental improvements, particularly in the elderly, following the use of HGH injections. One of the most famous of these studies was presented in *The New England Journal of Medicine* in 1990 by the late endocrinologist Dr. Daniel Rudman. Dr. Rudman firmly believed that the decline of HGH was a major factor in premature aging. To prove his point, he worked with 21 men from ages 61 to 80, all of whom showed advanced signs of the aging process, for a six-month study. Out of these 21, 12 were given HGH while 9, the control group, received a placebo. All the men were instructed to carry on with their usual lifestyle patterns—nothing was altered except the HGH ingestion. At the end of this study, those who received the HGH gained an average of 8.8% muscle and lost 14% fat.

It must be remembered, however, that there can also be side effects such as diabetes, hypoglycemia, disturbance of homeostasis, and disfigurement following improper use of the hormone. Many users do not achieve the desired effects. One of the reasons is that the body will slow or even stop its natural release of the hormone by increasing its levels of the anti-growth hormone somatostatin.

Evidence of this shutdown sequence was published in an article in 1988 in the *Journal of Applied Physiology*, which followed two groups of highly trained weightlifters who had no deficiencies of growth hormone. One group was given injections of the hormone, while the other group was given placebo injections containing no active substance. Both groups continued weightlifting throughout the study. At the end of the study, the group that had received the hormone injection showed a significant decrease in body fat with an increase in fat-free mass (muscle), while the placebo group showed no change. However, the study also revealed that the men receiving the hormone injections had a suppression of their natural growth-hormone response. HGH is not something to experiment with. The aid of an experienced physician is required.

Numerous companies have designed or are designing HGH-secreting agents that are called growth hormone stimulators (or potentiators). One class of these stimulators is referred to as the secretagogues (see Chapter 12). A secretagogue is a substance, chemical, or nutrient that helps to stimulate a gland to release a hormone. Some of the best and safest secretagogues available are usually composed of various mixtures of amino acids, including glutamine, arginine, ornithine, tryptophan, leucine, and glycine. These natural substances, if used under proper guidance, may presently be one of the safest and best ways to achieve higher HGH levels in the body. (See Appendix I for recommendations.)

Another class of stimulators work as actual growth hormone–releasing hormone analogs, which means they either mimic or stimulate the release of the actual hormone that releases HGH from the pituitary. There are some companies that are now offering a transdermal (through the skin) application for natural HGH stimulation. Whichever way you decide to increase your HGH levels, I would highly advise staying away from any products that contain actual HGH unless otherwise directed by your physician.

HGH and Fat Burning

As you will see in Part II, the human body relies on three basic sources of energy: carbohydrates, dietary fats, and dietary proteins. The carbohydrates must first be converted into glucose before the body can use them as an energy source. Excess glucose is converted into glycogen and stored, although the body can only store four or five hours' worth of glycogen. Once a good supply of the glycogen has been used up, the body begins burning fat. At this point, the body enters a semi-fasting mode. HGH is responsible for switching it into this mode.

> #### High Carbs = Low HGH
> If you are like most people and maintain high insulin levels throughout the day and evening by consuming numerous carbs, then your HGH levels could be low. Numerous studies reveal that high insulin levels negatively affect your body's anabolic (rebuild and repair) response by lowering your body's production of growth hormone.

HOW FAT IS TRANSPORTED

Blood is composed of approximately 50% red blood cells and 50% liquid. The liquid is called plasma. When the clotting factor (fibrinogen) is removed from plasma, what remains is called serum, a yellowish liquid that contains hundreds of different specialized proteins. The average person has approximately 3 liters of serum. The serum carries the essential, life-giving substances through the blood vessels to nourish all the cells in the body. The serum also carries the waste away from those cells so that they don't become toxic.

One law of chemistry is really quite simple: Fats and water don't mix. Blood and body fluids are almost all water. Thus, nature is presented with a problem: How to transport the lipids (fats, which include cholesterol) from one place to another? This is accomplished by a group of transport proteins called lipoproteins. Some are referred to as chylomicrons, some as low-density lipoproteins (LDLs), and others as high-density lipoproteins (HDLs). The density refers to the chemical protein content. The higher the density of the chemical protein, the healthier it is for us. Which means that some cholesterol (the HDL kind) is actually good for the body.

Albumin, the dominant transport protein in blood serum, is a very high-density lipoprotein (VHDL). In the simplest terms, the more of these fat-carrying transport proteins we have, particularly HDL and albumin, the better the blood is able to transport all the lipids, including cholesterol. Without these transporters, the fats would simply stick to the walls of the blood vessels and create havoc. Albumin has been called the life factor by many top researchers because the more we have, the healthier we are and the longer we live.

UNDERSTANDING ALBUMIN

Albumin has over 60 roles in the body, including transporting nutrients, removing wastes, maintaining cell stability, and controlling DNA replication. Albumin is also the major transporter of fatty acids. It has a special cargo hold for three fatty acids per albumin molecule, although it normally carries only two. Under stress, it may carry up to six. Albumin that is bound to correct types and levels of fatty acids is vital for cell growth. In the body, countless trillions of albumin molecules are continuously transporting fatty acids to and from cells and to and from the liver.

It is difficult to be fat, misshapen, and unhealthy when one has optimal levels of albumin. The average person has only 40 grams of albumin per liter of blood (with an albumin/globulin [A/G] ratio of only 1.5). Healthy people have albumin levels of at least 50 grams per liter (with a minimum A/G ratio of 2.0). Super levels are above 55 grams per liter (with an A/G ratio of 3.0).

Albumin Levels

Your level of albumin is determined by your level of immune/inflammatory proteins. The greater the stress on the immune system, the lower the level of albumin. Every single hospital in the world has attempted to raise albumin levels with high-protein diets, supplements, and even by intra-venous injection. In every case, this approach fails. Only by reducing the stress on the immune system, resulting in a natural decline in antibodies and inflammatory chemical proteins, can there be more room in the blood for albumin. The liver makes trillions of albumin molecules daily. When defense proteins rise (as when a bacterial intruder is sensed), the liver reduces production of albumin and less fat is mobilized. When these proteins decline, the liver increases the production of albumin and more fat is mobilized.

A New Approach to Personal Hygiene

Over the years, it has become increasingly evident that infections are the major cause of diseases that are linked to overeating or being overweight or in poor physical condition. Poor hygiene may also play a role.

Dr. Kenneth Seaton, an Australian research scientist who specializes in the areas of aging and immune function, has spent the last 20 years developing ways to enhance albumin levels naturally. Through his extensive research in this area, he developed a revolutionary system for cleansing the areas of the body that allow for easy entry of germs. Fingernails, nasal passageways, and the eyes are all areas that he focuses on. Germs and viruses don't just float through the air and magically attach themselves to us. Instead, they hitchhike into our bodies from these areas, causing immune mayhem and ultimately a reduction in albumin levels.

Dr. Seaton's clients have been able to achieve optimal albumin levels by following his easy-to-use system, which is called The Advanced Hygiene System. Higher albumin levels lead to improved physical health and a trim shape. Even hygiene has a subtle influence over physical condition and shape!

Check out *www.fatwars.com* for more information.

Although diet is of great importance for overall health, it is not the determining factor in the concentration of albumin. According to Australian researcher Dr. Kenneth Seaton, hygiene is the single most important factor. Hygiene determines the concentration of defense/inflammatory proteins. In simple terms, the stress on the immune system is a reflection of one's standard of personal hygiene and general health (such as whether or not one smokes or has chronic disease).

As you know, dietary fats and cholesterol are essential for life and good health. Because they are not soluble in serum, they require transport proteins such as albumin to get to the cells. The more of these transport proteins we have, the more we are able to handle dietary fats and cholesterol. People who maintain high levels of albumin and other carrier proteins can eat lots of dietary fats and not suffer consequences like deposits in the blood vessels. When necessary, they can generate lots of energy by efficiently utilizing the adipose tissue, quickly converting its fatty acids, and transporting those acids to the trillions of cells throughout the body. Without sufficient amounts of albumin, protein synthesis will fail, anabolic metabolism will switch to catabolic (breakdown), and you will not be able to lose an ounce of fat.

THE BIORHYTHMS OF FAT BURNING

The single most important factor in achieving fat loss, optimal health, and maximum life span is a slight reduction in overall dietary intake and an increase in energy production. I realize that this is not news. Although you already know this, pay close attention to the following paragraph. It could rocket you on to fat-loss success.

It is important to realize that the fasting period between evening and morning, if it's adequate, is probably the most effective natural way to cause beneficial secretions of HGH and its helpers, and to free the cargo holds on albumin. Nature has scheduled the optimal production of both HGH and albumin during the nighttime sleep/fasting mode. Optimal fat-burning/fasting periods usually occur from the evening meal (no later than 8 p.m.) to breakfast at around 7 a.m., approximately 11 hours later. Normally, during this fast period, the body switches to fat burning by around 1 a.m., provided the person goes to sleep between 9 and 10 p.m. and insulin levels are not elevated by any snacks along the way (if you must eat late at night, eat a protein-rich food). This fasting/fat-burning cycle is excellent for health, growth, repair, and slowing the aging process. Best results are obtained when this fasting period lasts for the full 11 hours. If we consume a high-carbohydrate breakfast, we can switch the body out of the HGH-producing fasting mode back to using sugars as the main energy source. Insulin will be produced, fat burning will stop, and protein synthesis will be interrupted.

The secret is simple. The evening meal should be no later than 8 p.m. Then drink only water (or an isolated protein mixture) until the first meal the next day, which shouldn't be rich in carbs. If you are able to follow these recommendations, you can profoundly reduce weight and improve health. And if you follow my advice in the exercise chapters in Part III and train first thing in the morning on an empty stomach, you can increase growth-hormone production and boost fat burning all day long.

KEY TACTICS

1. Change your preconceptions about fat loss.
2. Your genotype is fixed, but the expression of your genes (your phenotype) is constantly changing and directly influenced in either a healthy or unhealthy way by the foods you choose, your environment, and your lifestyle choices.
3. Hormones control how your body burns fat. You can control your hormones by what you eat.
4. Refined high-glycemic (insulin-raising) carbohydrates stimulate insulin, which in turn awakens the fat-storing enzyme LPL.
5. High-quality proteins stimulate the hormone glucagon, which in turn awakens the fat-releasing enzyme HSL.
6. Hygiene, overall health, and rest also contribute to your body's ability to burn fat.
7. Fasting from 8 p.m. to 7 a.m. is probably the most effective, natural way to help your body burn fat, while eating late into the evening is one of the best ways to sabotage your fat-loss success.

3

His Fat

Russell turned 50 almost a month ago, and he wasn't too happy about it! Then again, why should he be happy? Russell is not the man he was 20 years ago. Gone are the days when he could stay up all night and party with his buddies. Even if he misses a couple of hours of sleep, Russell feels it the next day, And gone are the days when he would proudly tear off his shirt on a warm summer day to expose a finely tuned physique. Those muscles have been covered with layer upon layer of fat. Russell wouldn't be caught dead taking off his shirt at the beach these days. Also gone are the days when Russell actually had enough energy to go to the gym after work. Now he feels drained when he gets home, mustering only enough energy to plop himself down on the couch. Exercise is reduced to pointing and clicking his new, high-tech remote. What about sex? What about it?!

Russell's temperament has also changed. This once patient and humorous guy now snaps at almost everything. Arguments have become the norm around the house—Russell's wife and children avoid him more and more. Russell has become what every man, woman, and child fears . . . a fat, grumpy, old man.

Russell is not alone—he's experiencing an all-too-common transition that is referred to as andropause. If the word sounds familiar, it's probably because it resembles that passage in a woman's life called menopause. (Andropause is actually called male menopause in some circles.) The word "andropause" first appeared in the literature in 1952 and is defined as the natural cessation of the sexual function in older men due to a marked reduction in male hormone levels.

Now, what do andropause and male hormones have to do with fat loss? Actually, they're the link between obesity and middle-aged men. Andropause works ever so slowly on unsuspecting guys until they wake up one morning as completely different people. The men we once knew are slowly replaced—by bigger, grumpier, flabbier ones.

IT'S MORE THAN JUST A SEX HORMONE

Just as menopause reflects a decline in a woman's hormonal cascade, andropause reflects a decline in male hormones. Collectively, the male hormones are called androgens. At the top of the androgen list is the one we've all heard of before: testosterone. Ninety-five percent of testosterone is made in the testes, and 5% in the adrenal glands. Testosterone is a fat-soluble hormone that is synthesized from cholesterol. It's the hormone that ensures the development and integrity of the genitals in males, but it also regulates the structure of all body proteins—and a whole lot more.

You thought testosterone was just a sex hormone? Wrong! Testosterone travels to every part of the human body. When naturally abundant, testosterone is at the core of energy, stamina, sexuality, and a lean body. There are receptors for testosterone throughout the body, from the brain to the toes. Testosterone is involved in the making of proteins, which in turn build muscle. It's also a key player in the manufacture of bone. Testosterone improves oxygen uptake throughout the body, revitalizing all tissues. This is important because oxygen is a fundamental ingredient in the formula for burning body fat. Testosterone also helps control blood sugar. Remember, excess blood sugar causes us to store fat at unprecedented rates, when the insulin that controls our excess blood sugar shuts down the body's ability to access fat as a fuel source.

After about age 35, a man's testosterone levels begin to decline. This slight dip in normal levels goes unnoticed at first and causes only modest changes in body composition—maybe a slight increase in those love handles from year to year. The decline in testosterone is felt not just in the tummy area. There is also a weakening of muscle strength and bone matter. Declining testosterone secretion also causes the organs to begin to lose their function over time, resulting in changes such as memory loss and increased irritability. A man will also notice more and more fatigue-related deficiencies. But it is the noticeable increase in body fat that will sound the first alarm that things are not as they used to be.

Restoring testosterone to optimal levels has been proven to:

- increase muscle mass (which sets the stage for a decrease in body fat);

- boost brain function, including memory, visual acuity, and concentration;
- protect the heart—it reduces virtually every cardiovascular risk factor (our number one killer, remember?), including high cholesterol, high blood sugar, abnormal clotting, and stress response;
- strengthen the bones;
- and, of course, lower insulin levels.

Testosterone and Obesity

The importance of testosterone can't be underestimated, especially in men who need to lose excess fat. Testosterone is an essential hormone for fat burning. An adult man's testicles normally produce 7–10 milligrams of testosterone per day. In over-fat or obese males, androgen (male hormone) levels decline in proportion to the degree of obesity—the lower the level of testosterone, the fatter the man becomes, and vice versa.

The hormone leptin, discussed in Chapter 1, is believed to be a major culprit here. Since leptin circulates in the bloodstream at concentrations in proportion to the amount of fat reserves, the higher the body's fat content, the higher the levels of leptin. But as men get fatter, leptin's message somehow becomes skewed and begins to inhibit testosterone production. (This may be one of the reasons why over-fat and obese boys often experience a delay in reaching puberty.)

The decline in testosterone goes hand in hand with the decline in muscle mass, which ultimately results in a slowdown in men's anabolic (tissue-building) metabolism. In the never-ending battle to control the slowdown of metabolism, adequate levels of testosterone are critical for slowing down the deterioration of fat-burning engines. You know the importance of muscle when it comes to fat burning—the gradual loss of testosterone that accompanies aging compounds the problem of excess fat by decreasing the amount of fat-burning muscle even more.

Swedish researchers R. Rosmond and P. Björntorp, in a 1998 study of 284 middle-aged men, discovered that low testosterone levels were indirectly or directly related to the amount of fat the men were carrying around their midsections. Those with too much fat around their abdomens were more likely to have major health problems like diabetes and heart disease. The Lipid Research Centre in Canada completed a 1997 study involving 76 men, showing that the higher the testosterone levels, the better the levels of good cholesterol (HDL) and the lower the levels of bad cholesterol (LDL). This same study showed that men with higher testosterone levels also had lower levels of triglycerides (the fats that travel around our bloodstream and are all too easily stored as body fat). Another 1998 study of 51-year-old men found that obese men were more likely to be anxious and depressed.

Testosterone and Exercise

In 1996, *The New England Journal of Medicine* reported on a study involving three groups of men. One group was given testosterone and prescribed a strength-training program, the second group was given testosterone and told not to exercise, and the third group did the strength-training program without testosterone. To no one's surprise, the group that exercised on testosterone gained the most muscle and lost the most fat, but the group that took testosterone without exercise had greater improvement in muscle and fat composition than the group that trained but didn't take testosterone.

There is a lot of research on the effects of proper exercise when it comes to raising testosterone naturally. The misconception is that aerobic exercise is the best exercise of all. The truth of the matter is that the only exercise that has been shown in studies to raise testosterone levels effectively is weight-resistant exercise. This does not mean, however, that you should avoid aerobic exercise altogether, as you will see in Chapter 13. When weight training is performed with a mix of aerobic activity, the benefits of each are greatly increased.

Testosterone in Chains

We certainly can't ignore the research when it comes to the fat-fighting potential of testosterone, but not all testosterone is created equal. Not all the testosterone in the body is biologically active. Since testosterone is a steroid hormone (meaning it's fat-soluble), it has to travel through the bloodstream on specialized serum-transport proteins. It is only the free, unbound testosterone and the testosterone bound to albumin (see Chapter 2) that exert their wondrous effects on men's bodies. The free testosterone is the most biologically active. So in effect, the total amount of testosterone that is made available to the body is only about half of the total testosterone in circulation.

The free, physiologically active testosterone is what declines the most with age. In a 1999 Belgian study involving 372 males aged 20 to 85, decreased levels of free testosterone went along with increased body mass index ratings and increased fat mass. The younger the subjects, the lower the fat levels and the higher the amounts of muscle tissue. This study also indicated that the younger subjects had much higher free testosterone levels than the older ones. Researchers concluded that free testosterone positively influences body composition.

Free testosterone declines with age because of a specific protein called sex hormone–binding globulin (SHBG), which binds with it. Testosterone is unable to do its powerful muscle enhancing/fat-burning work once it is bound to SHBG. It is not uncommon for free testosterone to decline by about 1% per year after the age of 40. In a 1998 Greek study involving 52 elderly men, it was discovered that the increase in SHBG was directly related to the increase in the age of the men. On average, there was a 13% increase in the transport protein per five years, making it harder and harder for elderly men to lose weight.

PUMP UP THE VOLUME!

The solution seems obvious: Men need to bring their testosterone levels back to what they were when they were lean and firm and happy.

Set It Free Naturally

Well, nature works in mysterious ways and can offer us a powerful alternative to artificial substances, which often have a number of side effects. I'm not talking about using testosterone injections to burn body fat. Instead, you can use what is already in your bodies and free that testosterone from the SHBG.

One natural herb offers us this potential without side effects—*Urtica dioica*, but you may have heard of it by its more common name, stinging nettle. Stinging nettle helps to release testosterone from SHBG; it also helps a man's prostate gland. In a paper published in 1995 in *Planta Medica*, an extract of the stinging nettle plant was shown to prevent SHBG from latching onto the cell membrane of the prostate gland and causing various prostate problems. According to this and other studies, stinging nettle extract is not only a powerful testosterone helper, but can also help to prevent and perhaps even treat prostate disease.

When it comes to increasing the fat-burning effects of testosterone, a particular extract of the stinging nettle plant is showing great promise. Special compounds in stinging nettle extract (known as lignans) have a very high affinity to SHBG. Researchers have been studying the beneficial effects of plant lignans on hormone-dependent cancers for some time now. These lignans are able to bind to SHBG in place of testosterone, and the bound testosterone gets thrown off the SHBG—freed to exert its physiological muscle enhancing/fat-burning effects on the body.

There are many different forms of stinging nettle available on the market, but it is only the newer extracts that are proving to be extremely powerful testosterone helpers. Many of the stinging nettle products on the market today have been extracted using alcohol or ethanol. These extraction processes either don't do an optimum job, or, in some cases, don't do the job at all. As you will note throughout *Fat Wars*, newer and better processes have been developed for most extracts; look for products that have either aqueous (water) or methanolic extracts. In this case, the difference could literally make or break the testosterone connection.

More on Stinging Nettle Extract

Stinging nettle extracts are also known to inhibit the enzyme 5-alpha reductase, which is responsible for irreversibly converting testosterone into the powerful metabolite dihydrotestosterone (DHT), and for inhibiting DHT from binding to the prostate. It is the DHT metabolite of testosterone that has been blamed for years by urologists for benign prostate enlargement. DHT is also a major culprit in hair loss on the top of the head.

Zinc is another powerful friend of testosterone. Not only is zinc an integral part of the enzymatic pathways that manufacture testosterone, but it also has the ability to inhibit the production of DHT.

Artificial Testosterone vs. Natural Testosterone

In Europe, a number of safe and effective methods of testosterone replacement have existed for years. Until the recent release of the testosterone patch and the newer topical delivery creams, the choices in the United States and Canada have been limited. Prescription options have been limited to taking the testosterone via injection or orally.

When testosterone is taken orally, it's rapidly metabolized by the liver, so injectable preparations of esters, which are more fat-soluble, were produced to ensure a longer life span in the body. Testosterone esters, which are more lipid-soluble, are injected in a peanut-oil base to increase the half life of the testosterone. One injection can maintain normal serum levels of testosterone for 10 to 14 days. These esters include testosterone propionate, testosterone cypionate, and testosterone enanthate.

Testosterone can also be delivered via testosterone patches and creams. Natural testosterone, synthesized in a laboratory (or at a compounding pharmacy) into an exact molecular duplicate of our own natural testosterone, can now be taken safely in larger doses by men who have a testosterone deficiency. I would personally recommend a natural bio-identical testosterone over other ones. These higher doses of natural testosterone seem to present no apparent health risks, as long as you follow the guidance of a qualified physician. You can easily obtain natural testosterone compounds with a prescription from your doctor through various compounding pharmacies in your area or through mail order.

These new pharmaceutical prescriptions include:
- Testoderm, a patch–delivery system of natural testosterone;
- Androderm, a similar preparation that can be applied anywhere;
- AndroGel (1%), a new dihydroxytestosterone gel that can deliver testosterone very effectively.

Testosterone levels naturally peak early in the morning. It is important to mimic the natural secretion pattern of testosterone in the human body when applying any patches, creams, or gels. It is also important to work closely with a medical professional for both evaluation and treatment with any form of testosterone, natural or synthetic, as it is a very powerful substance.

NATURAL TESTOSTERONE DISCOVERY

Elk velvet antler (EVA), an extract from an elk antler, is finally becoming known in the West. EVA has been used in Asia for over 2,000 years to treat myriad disorders. The extract is a living biological factory loaded with some of the most incredible substances in their natural synergistic ratios, including: amino acids, essential for anabolic metabolism; growth hormones, plus a whole array of growth factors and their precursors; and natural anti-inflammatory agents known as prostaglandins (most disease is associated with an increase in inflammatory messengers). Research reports on the benefits of EVA, coming from all over the world, are numerous, but one of the most exciting studies was performed in 1998 at the University of Alberta. This study showed that a specific extract of EVA, taken orally, was able to significantly boost the testosterone levels in the human body.

MEN ARE FROM . . . VENUS?!

As a man ages, depleted and/or bound testosterone are far from the only problems he faces. As men experience a drop in their testosterone levels, or a rise in their SHBG levels, they usually experience a rise in their estrogen levels too. In men and also in postmenopausal women, most estrogens are produced directly from androgens (male hormones). Androgens and estrogens have similar metabolic effects in the liver, where enzymes convert testosterone into estradiol, or E2, a form of estrogen. As men age, they lose muscle and gain fat, and the more fat, the higher the conversion of testosterone to estrogen. The less testosterone men have, the less muscle they make. It's a vicious cycle. In order to effectively reverse this cycle and increase the amount of natural testosterone in the body, men must also look at inhibiting this conversion of testosterone into estrogen. Once again, nature provides us with a number of powerful ways to help prevent this conversion from taking place. The following recommendations are all widely available at health food outlets:

- In addition to inhibiting SHBG binding, stinging nettle root has also been shown to inhibit testosterone-conversion activity.
- Soy isoflavones have been shown to inhibit conversion activity (but they also contain substances that act as weak estrogens that may be counterproductive in larger doses to the increase of muscle mass).

- One of the most powerful conversion inhibitors to date is a bioflavonoid called chrysin. Chrysin was shown to be similar in both potency and effectiveness to the estrogen conversion-inhibiting drug aminoglutethimide. In order for chrysin to become bioavailable to the body, it must be accompanied by an enhanced delivery ingredient, such as piperine (black pepper extract).

It is not uncommon for a man of retirement age to have higher estrogen levels in his body than a woman of the same age, provided that the woman isn't on estrogen therapy, so it stands to reason that the natural compounds available today to boost free testosterone may soon be a staple of any man's war on fat gain.

KEY TACTICS

1. The aging process predisposes men to gain fat in ways that become increasingly difficult to burn off.
2. Raising free testosterone levels is key for men to burn fat.
3. Testosterone levels can be increased through exercise, supplements, and pharmaceutical preparations (natural and artificial).
4. The loss of excess body fat with a subsequent rise in muscle mass allows the body to produce more testosterone.

4

Her Fat

A woman's body is designed to store fat. More than a man's?! Yes. Recent research has demonstrated that women's fat cells are different from men's in both look and performance. As a matter of fact, when researchers analyzed women's and men's fat cells, this is what they discovered:
- women's fat cells are up to five times larger than men's;
- women's fat cells can contain up to twice the fat-storing enzymes;
- women's fat cells can contain half the fat-releasing enzymes.

What does this mean? It means it's easier for women to put on fat and it's harder for women to take it off. This is not fair. In terms of evolution and survival, however, it is what worked. Evolution's priorities are not the same as ours. Women will have to work with what they've been given here. Obviously, women have evolved to ensure the survival of offspring, which requires a much larger reserve of body fat for sustenance in times of famine. Women have at least 8% more body fat than men have, which allows for an extra 120,000 calories for use in needy times. Nowadays, those 120,000 calories never see the outside of their storage containers (fat cells). Another difference between men and women: A woman needs at least 16% body fat to allow for proper hormonal production.

The odds in the Fat Wars are stacked against women from the start. We know that muscle is the metabolic engine of the body that causes us to burn fat. Men carry, on average, 40 pounds more muscle than women do. Men also produce 10 times more testosterone than women do—testosterone is a muscle-building, fat-burning hormone. Men manufacture up to twice the amount of fat-releasing enzymes that women do. The more of these enzymes, the faster fat is released as fuel.

All these factors give men a higher metabolism than women have. Men can burn, on average, 30% more calories during exercise than women can. To add insult to injury, men can burn, on average, up to 30% more calories while at rest.

AND THEN THERE'S ESTROGEN

Estrogen is a group of three hormones that regulate women's reproductive functions. Estrogen is also known to perform over 300 different functions in the body. It affects everything from building bones to strengthening the heart. Scientists now suggest that estrogen also works on regulating the brain. As I wrote in the last chapter, men's estrogen levels may actually increase instead of decrease with age, which is now thought to be one of the reasons that twice as many women are afflicted with Alzheimer's as men.

In women, estrogen is normally produced in the ovaries and, to a lesser extent, the adrenal glands. As women age, estrogen production from the ovaries and glands starts to dwindle. The body considers this decline in production to be a big deal. Over time, women's genetics have built in some clever ways to deal with this decrease. As the estrogen levels drop, the body is making plans for future estrogen manufacturing sites, and the best location seems to be Fat Central. That's right, estrogen can be produced in fat cells. On the one hand, this is a good thing. Your body needs estrogen. On the other hand, it is bad for your svelte figure.

A woman's body senses the need to start shifting estrogen production some time in her mid-30s. Now known as perimenopause, this is a period of very gradual transition that can last for up to 20 years—from the mid to late 30s for the majority of women, ending in their mid-50s. Perimenopause's ever-so-slight hormone changes affect a woman's cycle, including her mood swings and her weight. As Debra Waterhouse puts it in her book, *Outsmarting the Female Fat Cell,* "It is during these transitional years that a woman's body goes from that of an hourglass shape to a beer glass." Whoa!

Once estrogen levels decline to a certain point, fat-storing enzymes are increased and fat-releasing enzyme activity is slowed down or stopped altogether. The fat cells are getting ready to store, store, and store some more, so that they can become estrogen-producing factories as a woman gets older.

In case all this activity isn't enough to ensure sufficient fat cells for alternative estrogen production, women's fat cells also divide to create more fat cells. Fat cells only divide at select times in a person's lifetime, and perimenopause can be one of them. Yes, fat cells can split, ensuring that the body will have an ample supply of estrogen for the coming years.

LOCATION, LOCATION, LOCATION

In younger women, extra fat seems to find its way (no map needed here) to the buttocks, hips, and thighs much too easily. But as time goes by and a female's hormonal system declines, fat seems to become more preoccupied with one location.

The first thing a realtor is taught about real estate investing is that the better the location, the higher the returns. The female body understands the same principle, and chooses the tummy for storing fat because this happens to be the area most conducive to the production of estrogen. Fat cells located in the midsection insulate the liver and the adrenal glands, and it is with the aid of these two that estrogen is produced. The production assembly goes like this:

1. The adrenal glands produce a type of testosterone (yes, the male hormone).
2. The liver produces an enzyme that is necessary for the conversion of testosterone to estrogen.
3. The fat cells closest to the adrenal glands and the liver become the manufacturing plants for the estrogen.

All in all, it's a very sophisticated estrogen-manufacturing system that has evolved over millennia to ensure women's survival into old age.

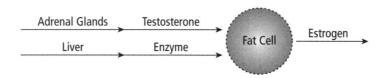

Figure 4-1: *The estrogen production line.*

To make sure that this manufacturing process goes off without a hitch, the female body does away with unnecessary metabolic machinery. After all, there's no need to burn fat when it's needed in larger quantities for estrogen production. To secure the fat, after the age of 35, the female body loses approximately one-half pound of muscle—the key metabolic engine of the body—a year. The loss of this metabolic machinery gives the female body the ability to gain at least one-and-a-half pounds of fat each year to replace the muscle. And, no surprises here, from her mid-30s, the typical woman often gains one-and-a-half pounds of extra fat each year.

I CAN'T STOP EATING!

Just because all that fat-storing capacity is in place doesn't mean that women have to take advantage of it. But wait! Another cruel trick of biology is about to kick in. Women seem to crave extra calories with increased age. Why is this? Because their declining hormone levels are wreaking

Women and Testosterone

Women need healthy levels of testosterone throughout their lives. Testosterone helps in their bodies' ability to utilize protein and manufacture bone mass. It improves oxygen uptake and helps control blood sugar. It helps regulate cholesterol and maintain a powerful immune system. Testosterone also appears to help with mental concentration and sex drive. If that's not enough, it improves mood swings by maintaining a better hormonal balance.

Normal levels of testosterone are especially important for perimenopausal and menopausal women. As women age, their production of testosterone drops or becomes bound to body proteins. The loss of testosterone shows in bone loss (osteoporosis), as well as in a loss of energy, libido, and muscle. One of the ways in which a woman can naturally increase her testosterone levels is through the action of another important hormone, DHEA (dihydroepiandrosterone). DHEA is the most abundant steroid produced in the human body. It is produced by the adrenal glands. And like many of the other hormones, it too declines with age. DHEA production reaches its maximum around 20 years of age. By age 80, women only produce about 10% of what they did at age 20. DHEA is a direct precursor to many other hormones, including testosterone and estrogen. This is the main reason why it has earned the nickname "Mother Hormone." So if a woman is low in DHEA, she will most probably be low in testosterone. By boosting their DHEA, women can help their bodies manufacture more testosterone.

Chronic stress is one of the main culprits behind DHEA depletion. DHEA is produced along the same pathway as stress hormones. During stress, cortisol—the main stress hormone—is seen by the body as the most important hormone. Production is shifted away from DHEA to make extra cortisol. When the body makes this adjustment often enough, DHEA/cortisol levels become out of balance and the immune and hormonal systems suffer.

You can easily obtain DHEA supplements from a health food outlet; however, since DHEA is a powerful hormone, I highly recommend a physician's guidance. DHEA levels can be measured by a simple blood or urine test, but make sure to check both DHEA and DHEA-S (sulfate) levels for accuracy. Youthful ranges of DHEA (measured in micrograms per deciliter) are 350 to 430 for women and 400 to 560 for men. Many people in North America (men and women) have levels below 100.

havoc all around. As the levels of estrogen drop below normal, the levels of certain chemical messengers in the brain also start to decline, including the key regulator of hunger: serotonin.

Serotonin is a neurotransmitter responsible for normal mood, behavior, and feelings of satisfaction. When serotonin levels are low, we feel tired, moody, and hungry. If we were hungry for vegetables, it wouldn't be so bad, but the hunger cravings are for sweets. The sugars from these foods can enhance the levels of serotonin, so to keep the brain happy, women eat and eat and eat until the brain is satisfied (which doesn't last for long). In the meantime, they've added more calories that they don't physically need—so those calories go into storage. (No doubt that was the plan.)

AND NOW THE GOOD NEWS . . .

There are benefits hidden in all this new fat—estrogen can now be produced to balance the negative effects of menopause.

Here's how the estrogen produced from fat cells helps women during menopause:

- it cuts the level of hot flashes to half of what leaner women experience;
- it allows for better sleep;
- it maintains natural collagen production, so skin stays healthy;
- it cuts the risk of osteoporosis to half the levels that thinner women face.

The larger a woman's fat cells become, the more estrogen can be produced. Research performed at the University of Pittsburgh showed that women who developed the largest fat cells produced at least 40% more estrogen than those with smaller ones.

The question is: Can women find alternative estrogen without having to pack on weight?

Estrogen Replacements

Even though women in Canada are much less likely to opt for estrogen replacement therapy (ERT) than women in the U.S., it still remains the most widely prescribed drug in North America, coming in at about 50 million prescriptions each year. The problem with these drugs is that they come mainly from a synthetic version of estrogen called Premarin.

Premarin is a blend of 10 various estrogens, of which only two are found in the human body. These estrogens are unnatural and are much stronger than the estrogen produced in a woman's body. (Premarin is actually produced from pregnant mares' urine, thus the name [*pre*-gnant *ma*-res u-*rin*-e].)

Estrogen's Buddy

If you're using estrogen replacement therapy, ask your doctor about prescribing natural progesterone instead of the synthetic versions referred to as progestins. Progesterone is a natural precursor hormone (like DHEA) that converts into various other hormones in your body, including estrogen and testosterone; as such, it should be taken along with estrogen. Research suggests that progesterone can help guard against uterine cancer. Your body can handle natural progesterone, whereas the body may have difficulty with the unnatural progestins.

While using ERT, some middle-aged women experience symptoms such as breast pain or breast swelling, fibrocystic breast disease, endometriosis, uterine cysts, bloating, weight gain, and depression. Many or all of these symptoms are associated with an estrogen/progesterone imbalance leading to estrogen dominance. Therefore, progesterone and NOT estrogen is usually deficient in these women. When the hormonal balance is restored by supplying natural progesterone, many (if not all) of these symptoms typically subside.

If a woman does not ovulate, she cannot create any progesterone. Understanding that women can have their periods without ovulating is important. Progesterone is normally responsible for preparing a woman's body for pregnancy and, if pregnancy occurs, maintaining it until birth by preparing the endometrium for a possible pregnancy, inhibiting the contraction of the uterus, and inhibiting the development of a new follicle. If pregnancy does not occur, menstruation begins. If pregnancy does occur, the placenta starts to secrete progesterone.

If you're currently on this form of estrogen, I highly urge you to talk to your physician about alternative sources of natural estrogens that compounding pharmacies will be all too happy to put together for you.

Here are two examples of natural bioidentical estrogen formulas that are available by prescription:

- Bi-Estrogen: composed of 80% estriol (E3) (the weakest estrogen) and 20% estradiol (E2);
- Tri-Estrogen: composed of 80% estriol (E3), 10% estradiol (E2), and 10% estrone (E1).

Studies confirm that the estriol (E3) hormone exerts a protective effect against some estrogen-dependent cancers, such as breast cancer, and that the stronger estrogens found in artificial estrogen replacements can sometimes increase a woman's risk.

THE PILL AND FAT LOSS

Women who use oral contraceptives may be limiting their success in the Fat Wars. Recent evidence uncovered by the Colgan Institute of Nutritional Science in California shows that the pill is responsible for lowered female testosterone levels. Remember, testosterone is needed to burn fat in both men's and women's bodies. Testosterone is also a key factor in gaining muscle tissue, and the more muscle tissue you carry, the greater your fat-burning reward.

ESTROGEN-MANUFACTURING PLANTS!

It may seem as if a woman's only choices as she ages are: gain weight to produce more estrogen, try to stay slim but be miserable, or pop estrogen pills. Well, all these choices sound pretty bleak—thank goodness for Mother Nature.

For millennia, women in Asia have stayed slim into their later years without any discomfort. How do they do it? They consume substances, such as soy, that contain phytoestrogens.

Phytoestrogens are plant compounds that contain estrogen-like molecules that have the ability to occupy the same receptor sites as our own hormones. "Phyto" means plant and "estrogens" refers to the ability of these plant chemicals to mimic the effects of estrogen in the body. There are already over 300 plants that are known to contain these substances, with many more likely to be found in this decade.

These phytoestrogens prevent the binding of more potent estrogens, all the while emitting weak signals to the body. These signals are between 1/100 and 1/1,000 the strength of the estrogen the body produces.

Phytoestrogens have been shown to protect the body in a multitude of ways, including reducing the severity of hot flashes, irritability, mood swings, and anxiety. They can also lower heart disease risk by lowering levels of the bad cholesterol (LDL), and in some cases they lower the risk of osteoporosis and breast cancer. As a matter of fact, Japanese women who consume these phytoestrogens have a whopping 400% lower risk of breast cancer than North American women have. Japanese women also have the longest life expectancy in the world, and are known as the healthiest women in the world.

Could it be that they just have superior genes? Perhaps, if it weren't for the fact that once these women adopt Western eating styles, they become just as susceptible to these major diseases.

A new study published in *The Journal of Nutrition* suggests that most postmenopausal women in the U.S. may be deficient in phytoestrogens. The study evaluated the phytoestrogen intake of healthy postmenopausal women in the U.S. and revealed that the average woman only consumed 1 milligram of phytoestrogens per day. Japanese people consume approximately 50 times this amount.

Our main interest is in one of the most exciting influences of phytoestrogens: their ability to help us lose fat. (Or help us not to gain it in the first place.) By eating some of these plant compounds, women may be able to reduce the amount of fat that enters their fat cells, due to the extra estrogen that the body senses.

Genestein

The isoflavone genestein is actually molecularly similar to the hormone estrogen, but it exhibits only 1/1,000th the activity. As a woman's estrogen hormone production declines (post-hysterectomy or during menopause), genestein can elicit a beneficial weak estrogenic effect (making up for some of the deficit). But when the body is experiencing an unhealthily high level of estrogen, genestein can, in some cases, help blunt the effects of the excess hormone by competing for estrogen receptors that lie on the cells' (as in breast cells) surfaces.

It is important to note, however, that when it comes to breast cancer some controversy surrounds this issue. Some evidence suggests that genestein (from soy) can help some women with high estrogen levels by competing for the same receptor sites as our natural estrogen, potentially reducing cell proliferation. Other evidence suggests that women with breast cancer who are low in estrogen may actually be increasing their risk of cell proliferation with added phytoestrogens like genestein. "These phytoestrogens could possibly potentiate the effect of estrogen in the body that can ultimately lead to more tumor cell growth," says Dr. Russell Graham, a naturopathic physician specializing in hormonal issues. It is best to seek your physician's guidance when it comes to soy isoflavones and certain hormonally related cancers.

Feeling Soy Much Better!

One of the best ways to incorporate this cellular insurance into your daily regimen is to consume more soy products, as Japanese women do. Soy products come in a multitude of forms. The most valuable are properly

fermented products like firm tofu, miso, or tempeh, which maintain their
essential phytochemicals. When it comes to the powerful effects of phytochemicals, the magic seems to lie in a class of compounds called isoflavones.
Soy contains many isoflavones, but the three that are most interesting so far
are genestein, diadzein, and glycitin. It is these isoflavones that have been
thoroughly researched and are responsible for soy's incredible powers.

Because the phytoestrogens and isoflavones are located in the protein fraction of the soybean almost exclusively, manufacturers have been
developing new technologies to isolate and create a new class of dietary
protein powders rich in phytoestrogens and isoflavones. Buyer beware!
Not all of these products are created equal. The quality of the soy protein
can make all the difference in its active isoflavone content. Many soy proteins are poorly produced, using an alcohol extraction method that
removes most, if not all, of the active isoflavones. Many mass-produced
soy products, including tofu, also lose vast amounts of their isoflavones
during processing.

The traditional Japanese process of fermenting soy foods preserves
their isoflavone content and even enhances the activity of the isoflavones.
When it comes to soy protein powders, only water-extracted soy protein and
fermented soy protein isolates will retain their natural isoflavone advantage.

When purchasing these new dietary protein powders, also make
sure they are certified non-GMO (non–genetically modified organisms).
According to the U.S. Department of Agriculture, over 57% of soy products
currently on the market derive from genetically modified soy. If the packaging doesn't list this important feature, it is likely from a genetically
altered source. Please read the labels! Without going into detail about the
possible future problems associated with genetically modified products,
suffice it to say that they are genetically manipulated to create greater yields
for the farmer. As a by-product of this manipulation, GMOs become highly
unnatural organisms and, as such, are less likely to have a chemical structure our bodies can deal with.

A Note of Caution About Soy

Although there are many benefits to consuming high-quality soy
and its isoflavone family, one must err on the side of caution regarding
its use by pregnant women, women with a family history of hormonally
related cancers, and newborns. Several animal studies in the U.S. and
Finland have indicated a possible risk associated with a high intake of
phytoestrogens during pregnancy and the postnatal lactation period.
These studies show a possible inhibition of the sexual development of
the newborn.

Approximately one-quarter of bottle-fed children in North America receive soy-based formula, which is more than is the case in other parts of the Western world. It's estimated that an infant fed exclusively on soy formula receives the estrogenic equivalent (based on body weight) of at least five birth control pills per day. By contrast, almost no phytoestrogens have been detected in dairy-based infant formula or in human milk, even when the mother consumes soy products. Until more research is completed in this area, please be cautious when considering the use of soy-based formulas and foods for your infant.

ESTROGEN DOMINANCE

Estrogen dominance refers to an all-too-common hormonal imbalance seen in middle-aged women and men in which healthful estrogens are pushed out of the way by unhealthful estrogens. Unfavorable metabolites of estrogen, referred to as "bad estrogens," include elements such as 16-hydroxy estrone and estradiol, which promote more active fat storage and increased size of fat cells. Alternatively, the "good estrogens," made up of the 2-hydroxy metabolites, support the mobilization of stored fat, making exercise more efficient at reducing fat stores.

New research confirms that hormone metabolism changes with age. As Michael A. Zeligs, M.D., a physician and nutritional expert from Boulder, Colorado, puts it, "Slower hormone metabolism in midlife can mean higher than normal levels of estrogen and a deficiency in its beneficial 2 hydroxy metabolites." It is these 2-hydroxy metabolites, deemed the good estrogens, that are able to support needed progesterone production in middle-aged women, protect against certain forms of cancer (especially breast and uterine), and help mobilize stored fat in both women and men.

The overproduction of bad estrogens (the 16-hydroxy variety) directly contributes to obesity. The 16-hydroxy estrogens act as an unregulated estrogen or "super estrogen," creating a particularly unhealthy form of estrogen dominance. Studies suggest that normal-weight individuals seem to have approximately three times more good estrogens than bad ones. So how do we increase production of good estrogen?

Dr. Zeligs has discovered that absorbable formulations of diindolylmethane (DIM), a phytonutrient from the indole family, provide the answer. DIM is found only in cruciferous vegetables: cabbage, broccoli, bok choy, Brussels sprouts, cauliflower, kale, kohlrabi, rutabaga, and turnip. Diindolylmethane has been shown in numerous studies to positively influence healthy estrogen metabolism by altering the enzyme pathways that produce a predominance of good estrogens (2-hydroxy metabolites) instead of bad ones (16-hydroxy estrogens).

Supplements with absorbable diindolylmethane actively shift estrogen metabolism to greater production of fat-burning 2-hydroxy metabolites.
The problem with most DIM supplements on the market today is that they
are very poorly absorbed by the gastrointestinal system. But Dr. Zeligs has
produced a patented, absorbable diindolylmethane that he calls Bio-DIM.

More can be learned about DIM from the Fat Wars Web site,
www.fatwars.com. (Recommended Bio-DIM supplements are listed in
Appendix I.)

KEY TACTICS

1. A woman's body is designed to store fat.
2. A woman's body uses fat cells to help manufacture lost estrogen
   through the transition into menopause.
3. Addressing estrogen deficiency through diet and supplements
   (such as DIM) helps replace lost estrogen naturally, replaces the
   body's need to use fat to manufacture it, and helps the body to
   burn fat more readily.

5

Baby Fat

Kids are not only growing up faster than ever, they're also growing *out* faster. Childhood obesity is reaching epidemic proportions in many developed and underdeveloped countries. Kids are taking their parents' lead and putting on the pounds of fat at an astonishing rate—and they're likely to keep those pounds for a lifetime. Obese teens have a greater than 50% chance of becoming obese adults. If they have an obese parent, the odds climb to 80%. Statistics show that more than 30% of our children are over-fat, and one in five is considered obese.

If you have a significantly over-fat or obese child, or if you are obese and are worried that your kids will follow suit, remember that the same conditions (and the same solutions) apply to both adults and children. The right foods, physical activity, and recuperation are the keys to solving the problem of over-fat kids. But kids are kids, and they need your know-how (and your good example) to help them make the right choices, which means they may need some strong encouragement from time to time just to keep them on track. Nevertheless, as a parent your main responsibility for helping your kids get on the right path lies in your ability to set a prime example.

The concerns are not merely cosmetic. The health of millions of kids is at stake. We know that being over-fat plays a huge role in the development of Type 2 diabetes. This form of diabetes used to be called adult-onset diabetes because only adults got it, but today there is an emerging epidemic of Type 2 diabetes in youngsters.

Aside from the obvious health problems associated with excess fat on our youngsters' frames, there are many self-esteem issues to deal with. Everywhere kids turn these days, they are inundated by images of their teenage idols with so-called perfect bodies. Have you caught a glimpse of today's hottest pop stars? Whether it's Britney Spears, Christina Aguilera, or the trio from Destiny's Child, they all have thin bodies, which many of today's teenage girls aspire to have. The problem is that when sights are set so high, genetics don't always want to play along and many a teenager feels left out. Too many teenage girls constantly complain about being "too fat," even when they're not over-fat at all.

CRP

A study published in the January 2001 issue of the journal *Pediatrics* looked at 3,561 U.S. children, aged 8 to 16. It's the first study to link childhood weight to a chronic type of bloodstream inflammation that, in adults, is linked to heart disease. C-reactive protein (CRP) is the cause of the bloodstream inflammation. Elevated CRP levels in overweight adults have been directly linked with the development of heart disease.

In this study, 7% of the boys and 6% of the girls showed signs of elevated CRP, along with elevated levels of white-blood-cell counts, another sign of inflammation. Dr. M. Visser, an epidemiologist who led the research, showed that overweight youngsters were three to five times more likely to have inflammation than their normal-weight counterparts. This study may also explain why overweight children run a higher risk of heart disease and diabetes in adulthood, no matter what their adult weight is.

According to an online poll conducted this year by Harris Interactive, a leading research and consulting firm, 17% of girls aged 8 and 9 and about one-third of girls aged 10 to 12 see themselves as overweight. These numbers compare with 16% for boys in the same age groups. Self-esteem is a huge issue for teens—it's tough enough in the world without being rejected for being overweight.

WHERE DOES IT BEGIN?

Nothing is cuter than a toddler being fed. The innocence of that toddler's face completely covered in whatever food you're trying to feed him or her is priceless. But the number of parents who think it's just as adorable to see their children eat anything and everything that's placed before them never ceases to amaze me. I have cringed too many times while countless parents have fed their kids pizza, cookies, cake, chocolate, and whatever else they could find to make their children giggle in processed-carb heaven.

When are we going to learn that it's up to us to teach our children the right and wrong way to eat? But the parental influence actually begins even before the baby is born.

The seeds for obesity can actually be sown in the womb. Fat cells can divide during the third trimester of pregnancy and have been shown to be very susceptible to increased insulin levels. Too much of the wrong carbohydrates during gestation can cause insulin to be secreted in response to sugars in the bloodstream. Studies have been done on mothers' blood sugar and the effect of elevated levels of glucose on gestating fetuses. Those fetuses whose mother's blood sugar had the highest readings became markedly obese children by six years of age. This had nothing to do with the mother's weight during pregnancy. In other words, pregnant women should be very careful with the types and amounts of sugar foods they consume, not only for their own sake, but also for the sake of their children.

Many offspring of mothers with diabetes have been shown to exhibit unusual patterns of fat growth:

- The baby is unusually fat at birth.
- The baby assumes normal weight by the first year.
- Fat starts to slowly accumulate on the youngster's body over the next several years.
- Fat accumulation begins to accelerate at year five (girls) or six (boys).
- By age eight, both male and female offspring of mothers with diabetes are considered obese according to medical standards.

Scientists believe that the mother's insulin is unable to cross the placenta and cause any problem in the developing fetus, but insulin itself may not be the problem. Insulin injected into pregnant women who are insulin-dependent has been shown to raise insulin antibodies, which do cross the placenta. Once in the fetus, these insulin antibodies are able to increase the rate at which fat cells expand and split. This and other research are showing the link between diet during early pregnancy and the effect it may have on fat metabolism later in life (being pregnant is not an excuse to eat everything in sight).

Over or Under: Which Is Worse?

Just as overeating and increasing carbohydrate consumption during pregnancy can set the stage for the child's obesity later in life, undernourishment during pregnancy may pose its own threats. A study of mothers who experienced caloric deprivation at a critical period during their pregnancies showed that they gave birth to children who experienced more than twice the normal incidence of obesity by the age of 19. Children whose mothers smoked during pregnancy were also found to be under-nourished, and similar numbers of them were obese by the end of their teen years.

Researchers once believed that an excessive number of fat cells in the young were only formed during overfeeding. This theory was disproved by a series of animal studies. In one of those studies, pigs that were under-nourished from the age of 10 days to one year eventually became very fat. These pigs had a normal number of fat cells at 10 days, but these fat cells were deflated, in a sense, and did not register by conventional cell count-ing at one year. But as soon as a good amount of food was supplied, the pigs' fat cells inflated like balloons, and the pigs became extremely fat. Not only that, but the longer the period of deprivation, the fatter they tended to become once it was over.

BOTTLES OF FAT

The baby formula industry is a big player in the Childhood Fat Wars, and it's not on the "Lean Team." The further away we get from our own nat-ural food source—that homegrown milk produced in the mother's mam-mary factory—the more likely it is we will flirt with obesity later in life. A 1993 study at Case Western Reserve University's School of Medicine com-pared rat pups that were fed a milk-substitute formula containing a major-ity of carbohydrates (56% of calories) with mother-fed controls who got milk containing only small amounts of carbs (8% of calories). The for-mula-fed rats became over-fat. It seems the source of calories, not the total caloric intake during the suckling period, can exert long-lasting effects on fat metabolism in later years, leading to the development of obesity.

Dr. K. Dewey and colleagues at the University of California found that the longer a mother breast-feeds and delays the introduction of solid food, the better the protection against adult obesity. According to their research, 95% of the obese had not been breast-fed. Breast-fed infants have been shown to be leaner than formula-fed infants at one year of age. Formula-fed infants were fatter because carbohydrates are much higher in commercial baby formulas, increasing the energy intake and causing an increase in insulin. So, early exposure to a high-carbohydrate diet may pre-dispose a child to over-fatness and obesity later in life.

PUBERTY PAUSE

Excess insulin and carbohydrate overindulgence in early childhood can affect our bodies later in life; one potential impact is the acceleration of the transition period between childhood and adulthood. Epidemiological research has proven that the average age of puberty in women has dropped

Ain't Got Milk

Our children have always been taught that milk is the liquid of champions. We were all taught that milk is good for us, from our doctors and nutritionists, and they in turn from the dairy industry. It turns out that we may be in for a big surprise.

Bovine (dairy) milk has been linked to childhood Type 1 diabetes. According to the National Public Health Institute in Helsinki, Finland, some pasteurized cow's milk (including many milk proteins) contains bovine insulin. It turns out that bovine insulin can cause the human immune system to turn against its own insulin production by forming antibodies that end up attacking human insulin. Therefore, according to this study, any child who is given cow's milk or formula that contains it may be at risk for diabetes. (Note: Buttermilk [found in whole milk] is the most saturated of the animal fats, containing a whopping 54% saturated fat. Buttermilk is also found in ice cream, butter, and fat-laden cheeses.)

Many studies have linked the consumption of cow's milk to such disorders as cardiovascular disease, bronchitis, asthma, pneumonia, diabetes, arthritis, psoriasis, lupus, and many immune-related problems.

It is important to note here that all cow's milk is not the same. Pasteurized cow's milk contains many antibiotics and hormones as a result of commercial farming practices to increase milk production. There are certain dairy farmers who do everything to keep the various antibiotics and hormones that may make cow's milk unhealthy out of their cattle. They are called organic farmers. The milk from organic farming practices may even contain a substantial level of a fat-burning fatty acid called CLA (more on this in Chapters 7 and 12), due to the natural feed the cattle grazes on. In order for optimal CLA to show up in milk, cows need to graze on grass rather than be artificially fattened in feed lots. Grass-fed cows may contain at least four times as much CLA as their non-grass-fed counterparts. Many dieters who consume milk tend to go for the skim (non-fat) milk variety, but unfortunately CLA is only found in the fat component of organic milk. If you are one of these "low-fat milk people," you may be depriving yourself of a very potent ally in the Fat Wars. So if you or your child insists on consuming dairy, try giving the organic variety a shot.

by four to six years in the past 100 years. A century ago, the average pubescent female was 17. Now, our little girls are becoming women between the ages of 11 and 13. Early teen sexuality, not to mention the risk of early pregnancy, are obvious social results. Obesity is another.

Obesity researcher Dr. Douglas L. Foster reported in a 1995 experimental biology meeting that the level of glucose (sugar) in our blood is the real culprit when it comes to the early onset of puberty. In his research, Dr. Foster was able to delay puberty in sheep by reducing the levels of blood glucose, and was able to induce early puberty by increasing the levels. The precipitous reduction in the age of puberty closely corresponds to the major increase in the consumption of high-carbohydrate diets in the last century. Many parents complain that their children, especially girls, are growing up too quickly. With the link made between a high-carbohydrate diet and early puberty, we now have another piece to the sugar puzzle.

KIDS AND FAT WARS

Early childhood is the most critical period for establishing anti-fat eating habits. What if a family has one over-fat child and two of normal weight? This doesn't mean the over-fat child should be deprived while the others enjoy unlimited French fries, colas, and sweet cereals. All children need to develop a lean and healthy lifestyle, and the battle must be waged as a family. If family members continue to indulge in fat-storing foods, do little or no physical activity, and burn the candle at both ends, all the kids will carry this behavior into adulthood. Sooner or later, it will catch up with them.

Pediatric studies suggest that obstructive sleep apnea, a respiratory sleep disorder that causes blood-oxygen levels to drop below acceptable levels and is characterized by snoring and interrupted breathing, occurs in approximately 17% of obese children and adolescents. It is theorized that sleep disorders in the obese may be a major cause of learning disability and school failure, although this remains to be confirmed.

Kids want things. They want the sugar-coated cereal they see on TV every Saturday morning. They want pop during recess at school. They want the munchie combo pack while watching their favorite movies. But guess what? Parents don't have to give in to their "I gotta have it now" cries. Instead of giving them what they want, give them what they need. Parents must teach kids and guide them into battle to save them from a life of obesity and poor health.

Notice how we're drinking more sugar-laden soft drinks than ever these days? Kids are especially prone to drinking high-carbohydrate drinks.

These "belly wash" drinks include not only pop (like colas), but also fruit drinks (juices) and other so-called "natural" drinks, loaded with added high-fructose corn syrup, sucrose, fructose, Maltodextrins, glucose polymers, dextrose, and the like. Insulin is working overtime to keep kids over-fat, and the sodas, chips, fries, and candy have got to go, replaced by (how dare I even mention this) water, nuts, and fruits like berries, apples, and oranges. Is it easy? No. Will kids gripe and whine? Likely. But like anything worth the time we put into it, we do what we've got to do for the health of our children.

Aren't We Going to Push Them over the Edge?

But what about eating disorders in adolescents? Won't your intervention just drive your kids to be so conscious about their weight that they'll go too far? The answer is no, so long as you approach over-fatness in children in a non-threatening way. You shouldn't be so concerned about weight; instead, focus on fat and how it influences their health. Over-fat kids are not genetic freaks. Over-fat kids rarely have a sluggish thyroid. Instead, they eat too much of the wrong foods, and they don't get enough physical activity. Concerned parents must feed themselves and their kids the foods that will awaken the fat-burning arsenals. Kids must be discouraged from doing too much sedentary activity, such as watching television, playing video games, or surfing the Internet. They must be encouraged to do vigorous activities that keep them on the move.

MAKING THE CHANGE: FAT LOSS FOR KIDS

Before suddenly turning a child's life upside down and charging ahead with a Fat Wars battle plan, it's important to spend some time with an over-fat child to map things out. Time and effort are required when making lifestyle changes. Fat doesn't magically appear overnight, so no one should expect it to disappear that fast either (I know that's not what you've been told on many an infomercial). It will take time to introduce changes into the child's life, especially with older kids.

Adolescents and teenagers need to play an active role in their personal fat-loss health plan right from the start. The first thing to remember is never place the child on a diet of reduced calories. A child's metabolism is especially sensitive to deprivation. When their cells realize that nourishment is being cut off, the fat-storing enzymes go into high gear. Then, when the child comes off the diet, their fat-burning enzymes, transport proteins, and hormones are so depleted that they easily put the fat back on, and then some. Sound familiar? Your mantra (and your child's) should be "Never diet, never diet, never diet."

LET'S GET PHYSICAL

Today's kids are less physically active than kids of earlier generations. Most children today catch a ride to and from school. In much of the world, gym class is a thing of the past. Many kids are brought up in a household with two working parents. In inner cities, playing outside can be risky, with an increase in crime, gangs, and traffic. For these reasons, many kids go straight home from school, lock the door, and turn on the TV. The hockey stick has been replaced with a video game joystick. The baseball glove has been replaced by a bag of chips. What can we do?

As parents, it's up to all of us to ensure that our kids, especially our out-of-shape, over-fat kids, are getting the proper physical activity that revs up their fat-burning engines by increasing muscle and forces them to breathe deeply and sweat. It's our job as parents to see to it that our sons and daughters get moving. This may mean joining them for a home work-out, finding a gym that has a children's physical activities program (such gyms are rare), or placing them in an after-school fitness program. Because the whole fitness thing may be new, some creative thinking on your part may be needed to make kid fitness work. It takes hard work, dedication, and ingenuity to make kids feel good about being more physically active. But rest assured, if you don't address your kids' level of physical activity, they are sure to fail to attain their fat-loss goals. Physical activity is an essential part of increasing their cellular activity. And an active cell is a fat-burning cell.

IF YOU FALL DOWN, JUST GET BACK UP AGAIN!

One thing I've noticed with many parents of obese children is that they hesitate to place their child in a structured sport, out of fear that their child will fall behind and be ridiculed by the other young athletes. This concern is valid. Organized sports can place great emphasis on winning and less on having fun, participation, and fitness. The over-fat child can be at a distinct disadvantage when playing sports such as football, gymnastics, soccer, volleyball, softball, hockey, and the like. However, this doesn't mean that the child is doomed to sit on the bench.

Over-fat kids, more than any other children, should be kept on the move. They need to be *more* physically active than other children because they have more to gain by losing fat and raising their level of fitness. A structured program is still necessary, but over-fat kids may need to get comfortable with their bodies and personal fitness before participating in any organized sports. Physical activity must always be fun and productive for them if they are going to get the fat-burning results they're after.

There should be good exercise programs available at their school. If not, it's likely time to create an awareness among the school faculty and the parents of other over-fat kids that there is a need for special physical activities directed toward over-fat or out-of-shape children.

A word of caution is in order, however. No child wants to be singled out—not a child with a learning disability, a physical handicap, or too much fat. A school-based physical activity program for over-fat kids must not look like it's just for the over-fat; otherwise there is a good chance that the other children will make fun of the participants. As a parent, you must build your child's self-esteem at the same time you build them physically.

> *Ryan is just 12, but he already is burdened with the responsibility of being alone at home after school until his mom gets home after work at around 5:30. This leaves Ryan with about two hours alone to do his homework, watch TV, and snack on juices, chips, and cookies. Ryan likes his snacks, and his excessive body fat shows it, but what to do? Ryan tried after-school programs, but since he was over-fat, he just didn't feel like he fit in. And the part of town he lives in is not as safe as it once was, so playing outside is risky. Ryan's parents prefer that he just come home and lock the door.*

Unfortunately, Ryan is not alone. He is, instead, one of an estimated 7 million kids in North America who are under the age of 13 and are home alone after school. Helping Ryan to improve his health and level of fitness requires careful planning. Perhaps families in the neighborhood can band together and form a play group after school, with stay-at-home parents taking turns interacting with the kids. Or when Ryan's parents arrive home, maybe the family can join in a group fitness program. The goal is to be creative and find a way to get your kids moving.

Television viewing after school may have to go. Research shows that the increase in television viewing, video game playing, and Internet use by kids has resulted in a rise in childhood obesity. When these leisure activities were cut back and replaced with more physical after-school play like tag, basketball, and climbing a jungle gym, the kids who were over-fat lost excess body fat and got healthier. Giving home-alone kids not only the responsibility to be by themselves, but also the responsibility for their own health and fitness, is a big step in the right direction. Parents must first set the example by helping kids see the light at the end of the tunnel. No one wants to see an over-fat kid become an obese adult.

KEY TACTICS

1. Obesity is increasing amongst children and teens in North America.
2. How we feed our children—whether still in the womb, toddlers, or teenagers—will affect their predisposition to obesity and over-fatness as adults.
3. Watch out for overly processed carbohydrates such as candies and cake and keep your children away from soft drinks. Reintroduce essential water into their lives.
4. The importance of establishing an active lifestyle cannot be overstated.
5. Lead by example.

Part II

Food for Thought

We all know that the foods we eat play a major role in how much fat we wear, but the question remains, exactly how does food make us fat in the first place? While the foods we consume contain a full array of micronutrients, such as vitamins, minerals, and enzymes, the bulk of our food consists of what are called the macronutrients: carbohydrates, dietary fats, and dietary proteins.

The macronutrients contain the energy (measured in calories, a unit of heat energy) that we use to help build and rebuild our bodies. They also replenish our energy stores, including muscle and liver glycogen (stored sugar) and fat (triglycerides). The carbohydrates and dietary proteins we eat each contain 4 calories per gram, while dietary fats contain about 9 calories per gram. Some foods, such as a sirloin steak, which contains a lot of dietary proteins and dietary fats, are obviously

more energy-dense than others, like a carrot, which contains carbohydrates and a lot of water. You pick and choose among these food options
every day. This brings us to what we all know about how we became
over-fat in the first place: We've chosen (and eaten) more calories than
we've used. Check out the following table, keeping in mind that an
active adult needs between 1,800 to 2,500 calories a day to avoid loss
of lean body mass. The more sedentary you are, the fewer the calories
you need.

A Global Comparison of Average Daily Caloric Intake

Country	Calories
U.S.	3,603
Germany	3,265
Mexico	3,136
Canada	3,093
Slovakia	2,892
Japan	2,887
Brazil	2,834
CHINA	2,734
Vietnam	2,463
Kenya	1,991

Most of us are born with the capacity to burn fat efficiently, although,
unfortunately, some of us are sluggish from the start. Other people are so
ready to burn fat that it doesn't seem to matter what they eat. As we age,
depending on how we treat our bodies, we can maintain a powerful system
that burns fat and keeps us lean or develop one that runs on sugar and
hoards our excess fuel. While genetics do control our fates somewhat, we
still have the ability to retrain our bodies to become fat-burning warriors.
Good foods at the right times will help to do this. It's not only the amount
of food that we eat that determines how over-fat we are; the type of foods
and when we eat them count as well.

For instance, I hear many health professionals tell their clients to consume more protein-containing foods from plant sources (this will be discussed in Chapter 8) rather than from animal sources (i.e., beef, chicken,
etc.). These people advocate the consumption of nuts and beans as sources
of protein. This is very misleading! Most nuts are very low in protein but
extremely high in fat (although some of this fat is actually good for you).

Beans (with the exception of soy) are also low in protein and are high in carbohydrates.

Nuts, Seeds, Beans, and Legumes	Fat%	Protein%	Carb%
Almonds (nut)	78	11	11
Cashews (nut)	73	11	16
Coconut (seed)	86	4	10
Pumpkin (seed)	76	18	4
Sesame (seed)	76	12	12
Garbanzo (bean)	11	22	67
Kidney (bean)	1	26	73
Lima (bean)	1	24	75
Soy (legume)	47	38	15
Split pea (legume)	1	26	73

In order to deem a food high in a particular macronutrient (protein, carbohydrate, or fat), that macronutrient must dominate the food's caloric value. Look at an example of a "high-protein" food like steak. The majority of commercially available (grocery-store purchased) sirloin steak contains only 29% protein, with the major macronutrient being fat at 71%. So in fact, most commercial beef is high in fat, not protein. But if you look at meat from a non-commercial, undomesticated source such as venison (wild deer) or elk, then protein becomes the major macronutrient at 82%, with a minimal fat content of 18%. This meat is indeed high in protein.

SIZE MATTERS

While we're on the subject of quantity, remember when a cinnamon roll easily fit into your hand? Not any more. Today the commercial muffins, cinnamon rolls, and sticky buns we find at the typical family restaurant are the size of softballs, with 450 calories each. In the land of plenty, we've come to expect a lot for our money when we eat at a restaurant. No fancy French food for us! We see a small meal come to the table, perfectly presented but definitely modest in size, and we ask ourselves, "Where's the beef?" Today we expect a lot of food, and restaurants are more than happy to give it to us. Super-size meals for super-size people. But what does "super size" really mean? It means more calories, more insulin, and ultimately more body fat. Even at more formal restaurants, we've come to

expect plates heaped with pasta, rice, potatoes, and breads. And what do we
do? We clean our plates.

In a 1999 study of 129 women, those who reported eating out the
most consumed, on average, 280 more calories each day than their dine-in
counterparts. That's a lot of extra energy, and it was likely tucked away into
their 30 billion fat cells. An interesting experiment set up by CBS Television
and the University of Illinois showed the level of gluttony we have become
accustomed to. During a movie matinee, each patron was given popcorn.
In Group 1, the moviegoers received a large tub; the patrons in Group 2
were each given a super-size tub. The researchers documented that the people who were given the super-size tub consumed 50% more popcorn than
those who received the smaller (relatively speaking here) tub. What does
this mean? It means that we will eat whatever is placed in front of us, without objection.

Not only do we not object to a large size when it's pressed upon us,
but when our turn comes in the fast-food line, we actually request it! We
all want the greatest value for our dollar. We look up at the menu board
and say, "super-size it." We choose the double-patty hamburger, the super
fries, and the huge soft drink containing enough calories and high-glycemic
sugars to rocket our insulin levels to Mars.

LIQUID CANDY

If you really want to drive lots of calories into your fat cells, then all
you've got to do is down a soft drink loaded with sugar, caffeine, and
phosphorus. Years ago, a soft drink serving was under a quarter of a liter.
Today, it's common to see cups holding more than a liter of pure refresh-
ment. But for some reason, we don't usually count sugar-laden soft
drinks as liquid body fat. We count the solid foods we eat, but don't give
the liquid candy a second thought. Kids who drink an average of 355 mil-
liliters or one 12-ounce can of pop per day consume 200 more calories
than the kids who don't. And since many kids drink pop instead of fresh
juice and water, there's a good chance that they're drinking a lot more
than 12 ounces of a beverage that is nutritionally worthless. How much
more, you ask?

A few years back, a report by the New York Hospital and Cornell
Medical Center's Nutrition Information Center stated that childhood obesity has as much to do with what kids are drinking as with what they are
eating. According to the study, between 1978 and 1994 the average
teenager in the U.S. consumed about 64.5 gallons of soft drinks per year.
Pop intake is implicated in a lot more than childhood obesity. In fact, there
is a direct link between excess soft drink consumption and calcium

deficiency (leading to bone fractures), tooth decay, loss of tooth tissue (enamel), and dehydration.

Our children are not the only ones consuming copious amounts of liquid candy. Another report from the National Soft Drink Association in the United States (yes, there is such an organization), entitled "Estimated Annual Production and Consumption of Soft Drinks," showed that in 1985 the average American gulped down the equivalent of 486 12-ounce cans of pop (that's 5,832 ounces of liquid sugar).

When you consider that the average soft drink contains 10 teaspoons of sugar (remember from Chapter 2 that you only need approximately 1 teaspoon to run on), you can see the mayhem your hormonal system is facing.

Liquid High

Many artificially sweetened drinks make people edgy, either from the sweetener itself or from the caffeine the drink companies are adding. If you don't think caffeine has an effect on our calorie consumption, think again. Caffeine is added to pop to bring us back for more. Numerous studies have shown that we will become addicted to pop in order to get just 100 milligrams of caffeine per day. Withdrawal symptoms are experienced for a few days when you cut back. The result is that no one withdraws—they just keep on filling up their liquid-candy containers.

> ### A Word on Artificial Sweeteners
> Throughout this section, I've warned you against the consumption of too much sugar, especially from soft drinks. This does not mean that you can just replace these liquid candies with artificially sweetened beverages. In fact, most artificial sweeteners can affect your health just as negatively as sugar itself (and in some cases even more so).
>
> These sugar substitutes didn't exist when our bodies were evolving over the last 100,000 years; therefore, our bodies don't know what to do with them, so they treat them as a type of sugar. A number of laboratory tests confirm that artificial sweeteners can boost insulin by actually fooling the body into thinking the sweetener is sugar. And remember, it's the insulin that causes your body to switch into a fat-storage mode. When your insulin is stimulated, it looks for sugar. When it can't find any real sugar from these substitutes, it ends up going after your own blood sugar, causing you to experience an energy decline and a fat-storage incline.

The ones to be extra cautious about are aspartame (Nutra-Sweet and Equal) and saccharin (Sweet 'N Low, Sprinkle Twin, and Sugar Twin), but I wouldn't recommend any artificial sweeteners unless the scientific evidence is conclusive regarding their safety (which it isn't yet).

The U.S. FDA and other health organizations have been bombarded with numerous reports about aspartame use being linked to seizures and many other problems, including dizziness, visual impairment, disorientation, ear buzzing, tunnel vision, muscle aches, numbness of extremities, pancreas inflammation, headaches, high blood pressure, eye hemorrhages, and more.

Caffeine withdrawal in children is very similar to adult caffeine withdrawal. Symptoms include fatigue, headaches, malaise, anxiety, and depression. The problem is further exacerbated by the fact that children can experience these effects after being without their liquid high for only a very short period of time, such as in missing just one or two of their usual soft drinks per day (i.e., at lunch or after school).

A 950-milliliter serving of one of the leading colas contains between 98 and 125 milligrams of caffeine, enough to get us really hooked. Kids may be at even greater risk because, although they weigh less, they can down a big drink as if it were water. Negative effects include nervousness, stomachaches, and nausea. If these weren't enough of a problem, the phosphates added to various soda pops increase kidney stone formation.

A U.S. Senate subcommittee investigated the soft drink issue in 1977 by gathering hundreds of pages of testimonies from leading health experts. After their exhaustive investigation, and seeing numerous problems associated with excessive caffeine intake, they recommended a reduction in soft drink consumption (no kidding, really!).

My recommendation to both you and your kids is to stay as far away from all sorts of liquid candy as possible. Learn to drink water instead. And especially be leery of the super-caffeinated sodas that companies have come out with over the last few years. These new ultra-high-liquid drinks can contain as much as 168 milligrams of caffeine per 12-ounce serving. There are just too many brands on the market today being targeted directly at our youth, so be observant and read labels. Better yet, try consuming more of what your body actually needs—water.

In the chapters that follow, you will learn about the various foods that contribute to your fat stores and the ones that help empty them. You will also learn why you're experiencing those insatiable cravings for the wrong types of food—cravings that are preventing you from losing your excess body fat. And I will show you once and for all how to control the triggers behind those cravings to bring your appetite into check. You will uncover the answers to why every diet you have tried in the past has not only failed, but made you a fat-storing machine instead.

Is There Any Good Sweetener Out There?

When it comes to safe and effective sweeteners, there is one I highly recommend. This sweetener will not cause a drastic rise in blood sugar levels and therefore is a good alternative for those with diabetes. It's called stevia extract. *Stevia rebaudiana* is a plant originally from the rain forests of Brazil and Paraguay. It's now grown in those areas, and in Japan, Korea, Thailand, China, and Canada. Stevia is between 100 and 300 times sweeter than table sugar (sucrose), but it does not appear to have any of the negative side effects associated with table sugar. It's very safe and widely used as a non-sugar sweetener in food and drink, and it is not broken down by heat, making it a great sweetener for cooking and baking.

As a substitute for those liquid-candy drinks, try adding fresh (and preferably organic) lemon or lime or a tablespoon of fresh fruit juice to a glass of mineral water. This mixed beverage not only tastes great, but is actually good for you. After two to three days, you and your children should be able to break free. Get the soda pop out of your life and begin the process of finally winning your Fat Wars.

In the following pages, you will probably see a complete contradiction of what you were taught about proper eating, a contradiction of what was and still is taught in our schools. But I will show you a better way to fuel your system, a way that will re-set your metabolic rate and, once synergized with proper metabolic exercise (which you will learn about in Chapter 13), will turn the Fat Wars in your favor. You're not going to call a truce here; after applying these principles, you're going to claim victory!

6

Macro-Fuel One:
Carbohydrates

Carbohydrates come mainly from plants. Grains, vegetables, and fruits are carbohydrates. Refined or processed carbohydrates also exist, such as flour and sugar. In order for foods to become usable substances in the body, their matter must first be broken down into its simplest form: molecules. In the case of carbohydrates, they are broken down into simple sugars like glucose—each carbohydrate food has an equivalent expressed as sugar. It's very important for you to realize that all carbohydrates eventually break down into sugar in the body. Whether you consume 1/4 cup of pure sugar or eat a baked potato, in the end they both become 1/4 cup of sugar to your body and your body will take the appropriate steps to bring its new sugar levels back into balance.

Does this mean that a baked potato is as bad for you as a 1/4 cup of sugar? Of course not. But in terms of your battle of the bulge, you must realize that your body can only deal with so much sugar at a time (1 teaspoon). Any excess will wreak havoc on your hormonal systems. Remember that winning the Fat Wars is all about balance. Through your food choices, you have the power to maintain that balance. If you are going to ignore what you've learned so far and eat a high-carbohydrate meal, don't be surprised when your mood goes from "I can do anything" to "All I want to do is sleep!"

Refined carbohydrates (and sugars) raise blood-glucose levels quickly and are the biggest contributors to high insulin levels. As you may remember from Chapter 2, elevated insulin levels are an over-fat person's nightmare. The body can't access fat as a fuel source when there are high levels of insulin floating around. And a very large percentage of people, especially over-fat people, have high resting insulin levels most, if not all, of the time. In fact, over-fat people have high insulin levels not only in their blood, but also in their cells, creating a sluggish metabolism.

The overflow of insulin has been proven to spell the end to fat-loss goals and, in the process, cause a lot of destruction. In a 1996 experiment, people were given substances to increase their insulin- and blood-sugar levels, plus an infusion of various fatty acids. The experiment showed that both glucose and insulin determine how effectively fat gets burned as fuel: High glucose/insulin levels reduced the concentration of the enzyme that transports fatty acids for burning to 45% of its normal level.

The high-carbohydrate diet creates a vicious circle. At the muscle cell level, years of poor diet, likely combined with a lack of exercise (the technical name for which is hypokinesis) and stress, have caused the muscle cells to go flat. Over-carbed and under-worked muscle cells just don't function as they should—they're like a stagnant pond that's practically devoid of life. So not only is there an oversupply of blood sugar, but it also can't get into the flat muscle cell; it's floating around in the bloodstream with no place to go.

An alarm rings out in the pancreas: Pump out more insulin—NOW! For hours, perhaps all day, insulin is elevated to deal with this blood sugar onslaught. As you are now well aware, this stops fat burning cold. In fact, it jams a great amount of the meal right into your 30 billion fat cells. You know the saying, "Might as well apply it directly to my hips"? Nothing burned, everything gained.

This high insulin will not be detected by the standard blood-sugar tests that are performed in a routine checkup. You won't have high blood-sugar levels as long as the pancreas is pumping out lots of insulin (hyperinsulinemia) and eventually bullying the sugar into the cells. As far as the blood-sugar test is concerned, everything is cool—no diabetes here. You already know that insulin makes you fat. But high insulin levels also cause damage to the cardiovascular system by promoting the division of arterial smooth muscle cells, thus stimulating plaque formation. This excess division of the cells that line our arteries causes our blood vessel walls to narrow and accumulate a build-up of sludge. Various deposits of cholesterol and calcium are attracted to the arteries, eventually creating what medical science calls atherosclerosis.

A study published in Germany in 2000 showed that people with Type 2 diabetes and impaired glucose tolerance were at a significantly greater risk for atherosclerosis. People with diabetes who inject insulin typically develop clogging of the arteries (atherosclerosis) up to 20 years earlier than their non-injecting counterparts. This information should be a wake-up call if you've been allowing high insulin levels to create a potentially hazardous situation to your cardio system.

In the case of people with cardiovascular disease, there is an excellent chance that they have high insulin levels, too, and excess carbohydrate consumption does much more than just raise insulin levels and cause us to gain fat. Overindulgence in the wrong kinds of carbs also raises blood triglyceride and cholesterol levels.

The reason why 95% of all people with Type 2 diabetes are over-fat is that they have had high insulin levels over a long period of time—their pancreases were pumping it out to combat the excess blood sugar. Eventually, the cells went from working poorly with insulin to becoming insulin resistant. The result? Type 2 diabetes.

> ### I Hear You Knocking, but You Can't Come In
> Many dietary endocrinologists believe that up to three-quarters of the people in the world are physiologically unable to handle a high-carbohydrate diet.
>
> If you are one of these people and you continually eat highly processed foods, then you will most likely develop insulin resistance. The insulin receptors that are responsible for transporting the excess glucose from the bloodstream become ever-more resistant to opening their doors and allowing the glucose to enter. Over time, this creates a situation where even small amounts of sugar can lead to high blood-glucose levels—the term for which is glucose intolerance. As cells become more and more resistant to hearing insulin's knock on the door, insulin has no alternative but to bust down the doors, bullying the cells into accepting glucose by increasing its levels until the job is done. This leads to hyperinsulinemia—a condition caused by insulin resistance.

SIMPLY COMPLEX

The carbohydrates we eat that get turned into blood sugar much too fast are another enemy in the Fat Wars. For a long time, researchers thought that simple sugars (refined) entered the bloodstream faster than any other sugars, but in the 1980s some Australian and Canadian pioneers in the field of carbohydrate and blood-sugar research discovered otherwise. Those complex carbohydrates we had worshiped as the bastions of health—the breads, potatoes, pasta, and rice (white) we consumed as the staples of our diets—were actually raising insulin levels through the roof, even more so than some simple carbs.

Today, many carbohydrate-rich foods are ranked according to how fast they get into the bloodstream, on a scale from 0 to 100 called the glycemic index. The index measures the speed at which the carbohydrates break down and put sugar into the bloodstream. Some break down quickly during digestion, causing a drastic rise in blood-sugar levels. These have the highest glycemic index rating. Glucose, at a dose of 50 grams, is used as the benchmark and is given a rating of 100 because it raises blood sugar super-fast. Other carbohydrates are ranked in relation to glucose. The glycemic index measures how much your blood glucose increases over a period of two or three hours after a meal.

Dr. David Jenkins, professor of nutrition at the University of Toronto, was the first to develop the concept of the glycemic index to help determine which foods are best suited for people with blood-sugar disorders (diabetes). In 1981, Dr. Jenkins released a groundbreaking study called "Glycemic Index of Foods: A Physiological Basis for Carbohydrate Exchange." In the subsequent 15 years, hundreds of clinical studies in the United Kingdom, France, Italy, Canada, and Australia have proved the value of the glycemic index.

To develop a glycemic index rating for a particular carbohydrate, 50 grams of the food is consumed and then the subject's blood-sugar level is measured. If the carbohydrate raises blood sugar quickly, it's given a high number on the glycemic index. It is the high-glycemic carbohydrates that you should consume less of. They overstimulate insulin production, which reduces calorie burning (and harms the pancreas and heart). Low-glycemic carbs can help keep insulin levels low so that more calories can be burned up instead of stored.

A selected list of carbohydrate foods, grouped by their respective glycemic ratings, is shown in the Fat Wars Glycemic Index later in this chapter. This is a relatively small list, and there are obviously many more foods to consider, but it gives a good indication of which foods to consume and which ones to cut back on (or avoid altogether). Many favorite foods, including some you've been told are good diet foods, are actually in the highest group on the glycemic index. Master the glycemic index and you'll be better able to sort enemies from allies in the Fat Wars.

Just because a food has a higher glycemic index rating doesn't mean that you should avoid it entirely. You can combine a small amount of a high-glycemic food with a quantity of low-glycemic foods and get a balance. Foods like carrots, which have a fairly high rating, are fine in moderation. Remember that a carrot is full of water, and you would have to eat a half-dozen carrots to get a significant boost. Calorie-dense carbohydrates like breads, pastas, rice, and potatoes must be eaten in moderation (especially during the 45-day transformation period). It's also important to realize that how a food is cooked will affect its glycemic rating. For example, pasta cooked al dente takes longer to break down while being digested than soft pasta. Usually the longer a food is cooked, the more quickly it will break down into sugars.

THE FAT WARS GLYCEMIC INDEX

The following foods are grouped according to their rating on the glycemic index. The best carbohydrate choices are in the low-glycemic group within the index. Restock the refrigerator and pantry to emphasize low-glycemic foods. Ditch the refined breads and breakfast cereals, baked and mashed spuds, white rice and rice cakes, toaster waffles, tater tots, and French fries. The consumption of high-glycemic foods spikes insulin and reduces glucagon, thus preventing the burning of body fat. Any high-glycemic foods should only be consumed in minimal quantities and should be combined with dietary proteins and fats in a meal. But remember, even too much of the low-glycemic foods can make you over-fat.

At first glance, eating according to the Glycemic Index may seem a little restrictive. If this is so, you have to ask yourself what you've come to rely on as the basis for sound nutrition. The answer will probably be man-made, pre-prepared high-glycemic foods. By preparing your meals around the Fat Wars Glycemic Index, you will not only be learning to eat the right foods for proper hormonal health, energy, and fat loss, but you'll also be developing tasty meals in the process. Giving up an old habit is never easy at first, but over time, when you've experienced the benefits of this new way of eating, you will never want to return to your old ways.

LOW-GLYCEMIC FOODS: Rated 20–49 (Allies)

FRUITS:

• Apples	• Apricots
• Berries	• Cherries
• Grapefruit	• Oranges
• Peaches	• Pears
• Plums	• Strawberries

VEGETABLES:

• Artichokes	• Asparagus
• Adzuki beans	• Black beans
• Black-eyed peas	• Bulgur
• Butter beans	• Celery

- Garbanzo beans
- Navy beans
- Peppers
- Split peas

- Lettuces
- Peanuts
- Soybeans
- Tomatoes

GRAINS:
- Barley
- Muesli cereal
   (without dried fruit)
- Whole grain pastas

- Bran cereals
- Whole grain breads
- Wild rice

DAIRY:
- Low-fat cottage cheese
- Organic plain yogurt
   (no added sugar)

- Organic milk

BEVERAGES:
- Fresh vegetable juice
- Green tea
- Water

- Grapefruit juice
- Tomato juice

SWEETENERS:
- Fructose (not recommended)
- Stevia

- FOS (frycto-oligo-saccharides)

**MODERATE-GLYCEMIC FOODS: Rated 50–69
(Limit Consumption)**

FRUITS:
- Grapes
- Mangos
- Watermelons

- Kiwis
- Pineapples

VEGETABLES:
- Beets
- Corn on the cob
- Onions
- Potatoes (red, white)
- Sweet potatoes

- Carrots
- Lima beans
- Peas
- Potato chips
- Yams

GRAINS:
- Basmati rice
- Buckwheat
- Oatmeal
- Pita bread
- Pumpernickel bread
- Whole wheat bread
   (100% stone-ground)

- Brown rice
- Cereal (low sugar)
- Most pastas
- Popcorn
- Sourdough bread

DAIRY:
• Custard

BEVERAGES:
• Apple juice
• Blueberry juice
• Black cherry juice
• Orange juice

SWEETENERS:
• Barley malt
• Organic unrefined
  brown sugar
• Unrefined raw honey
• Organic grade-C maple syrup
• Unprocessed blackstrap
  molasses

**HIGH-GLYCEMIC FOODS: Rated 70–100
(Eat At Your Own Risk)**

FRUITS:
• Bananas (ripe)
• Raisins
• Papayas

VEGETABLES:
• Cooked carrots
• Parsnips
• Sweet corn
• French fries
• Potato (baked)

GRAINS:
• Bagels
• Corn chips
• Rice cakes
• Doughnuts
• Hamburger and
  hotdog buns
  Pancakes
• Puffed rice or wheat
• Toaster waffles
• White rice
• Whole wheat bread
• Breakfast cereals (refined with
  added sugar)
• Corn flakes
• Crackers and crispbread
• French bread
• Muffins (due to the
  processed flour)
• Pretzels
• Shredded wheat
• White bread

DAIRY:
• Ice cream

BEVERAGES:
• Carrot juice
• Soft drinks and sport drinks
  (added sugars)

SWEETENERS:
• Corn syrup solids
• High-fructose corn syrup
• Maltose
• Sucrose (table sugar)
• Glucose and glucose polymers
  (Maltodextrin-based drinks)
• Honey

CHOOSING CARBS THE GLYCEMIC WAY

One trick to keeping blood sugar low and insulin in check is to eat like a caveman. That is, eat like we did when all we had access to were natural, unprocessed foods. The foods at the bottom of the food chain—the unprocessed fruits (especially from the berry family) and vegetables that are high in fiber and water—are among the lowest on the glycemic index. In contrast, highly processed foods—the ones we either "improved" or that are completely artificial—like white pasta and breads are among the highest.

The Problem with Sucrose

Out of all the sweeteners in the world, nothing seems to contribute to obesity more than good old table sugar (sucrose). It is a very hard sugar for your body to handle, due to the minerals that are needed to digest it, such as chromium, manganese, cobalt, copper, zinc, and magnesium. These happen to be the very minerals that are stripped from sugar during the refining process. As a result, sugar depletes the body's own mineral reserves as it gets metabolized.

The negative effects of sucrose are due to its molecular structure, one glucose molecule bonded to one fructose molecule. It is the fructose portion that seems to cause the most problems. In both human and animal studies, fructose infusion has been shown to cause a large decrease in liver ATP levels—ATP is our bodies' most important energy molecule. Losing any significant quantity of ATP could cause major health problems. And since the liver uses at least 12% of the entire ATP supply the body makes each day, a drop in ATP can spell disaster to the body's ability to detoxify properly, causing a build-up of toxins.

The powerful combination of glucose and fructose—such as you find in table sugar—stimulates your insulin more than anything else tested. So STAY AWAY FROM REFINED TABLE SUGAR at all costs if you want to lose body fat and maintain or gain back your health.

The worst of the high-glycemic carbs are scattered like land mines all around you in the form of fat-free snacks. Fat-free doesn't mean calorie-free and, more often than not, it means high glycemic. When in doubt, check the Fat Wars Glycemic Index and eat the foods in the first group (with a rating below 50) as much as possible. Whole books are available about the glycemic index, which contain big tables with dozens of foods listed. These tables will likely grow in the future as more people become interested in the glycemic index. For a printable detailed version of the glycemic index, see *www.fatwars.com*.

While the Fat Wars Glycemic Index is very useful when selecting carbohydrate foods, it's not designed to be the only guide to the way you should eat. You should also take into consideration the overall amount of macronutrients you ingest. After all, carbohydrates are not the only things that can make us fat. Overconsumption of calories in general will also pack on the extra layers. The amount and kinds of fats, dietary proteins, and fiber and the overall nutritional value of the foods you consume are also of paramount importance. French fries and potato chips have a lower glycemic rating than a baked potato, but the type of dietary fat they contain doesn't make them a great food choice. (A piece of cardboard also has a low glycemic rating, but this isn't a good reason to eat it.)

The percentage of carbohydrates in your daily diet can play a key role in health and burning body fat (more on this in Part III), provided they are low glycemic, fresh, unprocessed (as much as possible), and packed with phytonutrients and fiber. Research shows that when a high-carbohydrate diet is replaced with one containing more protein, the benefits include lower blood fats (triglycerides and LDL cholesterol), reduced insulin, and an increase in fat burning. Make sure the carbohydrate portion of your meals is rich in complex low-glycemic fresh vegetables and fruits, and low in simple (refined) high-glycemic ones like grains and processed cereals.

Low-Glycemic Facts:
- Low-glycemic foods do not stimulate food-craving hormones.
- Low-glycemic food plans are not based on starvation or deprivation.
- Low-glycemic food plans have been proven to reduce the incidence of Type 2 diabetes and to help control Type 1 and Type 2 diabetes, hypoglycemia, and hypertension.
- High-glycemic foods elevate insulin and blood glucose, stimulate fat storage, exacerbate hyperactivity, and reduce sports performance. Low-glycemic foods do not.

KEY TACTICS
1. Carbohydrates are converted to sugar in the body, which boosts insulin and inhibits fat loss.
2. Some carbohydrates are converted to sugar at unacceptable rates in the Fat Wars.
3. Consult the Fat Wars Glycemic Index for the right foods to eat. Only consume foods from the low to moderate lists in order to ensure fat-loss success.
4. Stay away from sucrose (table sugar) and high-fructose corn syrup at all costs.
5. Eat like a caveman.

7

Macro-Fuel Two:
Dietary Fats

Dietary fats (fatty acids) don't always make us fat. In fact, some fats actually help us lose unwanted body fat. Over the last 20 years, we have seen low-fat diets hit the market in a big way, leading us to believe that if we replaced fat-laden foods with low-fat (or no-fat) foods, our problems would be solved. Because dietary fat has 9 calories per gram, compared with 4 calories per gram of carbs, we assumed that if we just reduced our consumption of dietary fats and raised our consumption of carbohydrates, we would lose fat.

Unfortunately, it's not that simple. You can easily see this when you consider how livestock such as cattle are prepared for slaughter. In order to fatten them up as much as possible, they're stuffed into crowded feedlots, allowed almost no activity, and fed all the high-glycemic grain (containing 90% carbohydrates) they can possibly eat. Once again, carbohydrates come out the winner in the Fat Wars.

Over the last decade, we've become even fatter, with nearly 30% more of us moving into the obese category. High-glycemic carbs are not the answer to our fat-burning woes. Elimination of dietary fats is not the answer either. Fat consumption is okay—it's just that the wrong type of dietary fats can turn muscle cells into lousy fat burners. Many research studies show that if we keep our "good" dietary fat consumption within the range of 20% to 35% of total food intake, it will not make us fat. In fact, as you will find out in this chapter, we can't live without fat. Even prestigious organizations such as the Canadian Heart and Stroke Foundation and the American Heart

Association now suggest that we should be consuming up to 30% of our calories from the right types of fats (more on this later).

Too many people have tried cutting all the fat from their diets, only to find, to their amazement, that instead of the fat magically disappearing, they had an even harder time losing it. It is this unwarranted fear of fats or "fat phobia" that has led to our overwhelming carbohydrate indulgence of the last 20 years. When you restrict fat intake, not only do you limit beneficial fatty acids that are needed by every cell of the body, but you end up restoring the caloric deficit with extra carbohydrates (usually of the high-glycemic variety). Therefore, most low-fat diets are actually high-carbohydrate diets in disguise.

CUTTING THE FAT

What really happens to your body when you decide to cut out most of the fats from your diet and replace them with extra carbohydrates? This question was answered during a study at Rockefeller University in New York. Normal-weight people were placed on either a 40% fat diet or a 10% fat diet and checked every 10 days to see how much fat they were making. Yes, the body is very good at making FAT from CARBOHYDRATES (as covered in Chapter 2). Those on the high-fat diet were making little or no fat, as measured by triglyceride levels and triglyceride content. Those on the low-fat diet, however, were having a very different reaction. Doctors discovered that between 30% and 57% of the fatty acids in the bloodstream was saturated fat *manufactured* by the body. In short, those eating low-fat, high-carbohydrate diets *made more of their own saturated fat*!

Genetically we haven't changed much from thousands of years ago when we consumed wild game, fish, and nuts. How were these foods different from the foods of today? Not only were they low glycemic, but they also contained good amounts of friendly fats. Today, our diets have a totally different dietary fat content from the ones we were genetically made for, which is why we suffer from many unfriendly fat-related diseases, including cardiovascular disease, arthritis, diabetes, hypertension, and obesity, just to name a few.

SEPARATING THE FAT ALLIES FROM THE FAT ENEMIES

Dietary fats are essential to life; it's the type of fat you eat that can make all the difference in the world. Natural whole foods contain dietary fats as part of their structural components, and have a balance of saturated fats, monounsaturated fats, and polyunsaturated fats. The wrong fats, like trans fats, or too much saturated fat from animal products, can cause your fat-burning muscle cells to become sluggish and lazy. As long as you don't overdo your consumption of dietary fats, and you eat the right kind, you can gather fat allies in the Fat Wars.

Dietary fats and the fat that lines our bodies (body fat) are made up of combinations of one to three fatty acids with a glycerol molecule (which is actually an alcohol). These fats, depending on the number of fatty acids, are mono-1 fatty acid, di-2 fatty acid, or tri-3 fatty acid glycerides. The structure or chemical composition of the fat molecule is what decides its degree of saturation. Each is made up of a chain of carbon atoms with hydrogen atoms attached. The type of dietary fat (and how it works with the rest of the body's chemistry) is determined by the length of the carbon chain, as well as the number of double bonds and the arrangement of the hydrogen atoms that are attached. Most dietary fats contain mixtures of monounsaturated, polyunsaturated, and saturated, with one predominating.

Saturated Fat

A saturated fat is simply a dietary fat with single bonds (-) between all the carbon atoms (C) and no hydrogen vacancies. This means that the carbon chain is carrying its maximum number of hydrogen atoms. These fats are vital to our biochemistry, but our bodies can usually manufacture all that they need from raw materials (food). Saturated fats have a molecularly straight structure that allows them easy access into our already bulging fat cells (like arrows entering a bull's-eye). In essence, they are only useful as fuel, and no one has to remind us of how much extra fuel we are already carrying. They are found in high concentrations in meat and dairy products. In excess, they contribute to obesity, cardiovascular disease, certain cancers, and insulin insensitivity.

By limiting consumption of saturated fats, you'll improve muscle cell activity, increase your fat-burning rate, and reduce the deposit of fatty acids into your fat cells. (High saturated fats combined with low-fiber diets are even worse; they are associated with high insulin levels leading to over-fatness, obesity, and pre-diabetic conditions.) Saturated fats are found in all animal fats, dairy products, coconut oil, cocoa butter, palm oil, and kernel oil. Kernel oil contains special antioxidants and coconut oil also contains medium-chain fatty acids that the body mostly uses as an energy source, so if you're going to consume saturated fats, these two choices are your best ones.

Villain or Hero?

To set the record straight, it is important to note that not all saturated fats are the bad guys we've been led to believe. Dr. Mary Enig, author of *Know Your Fats: The Complete Primer for Understanding the Nutrition of Fats, Oils and Cholesterol*, is one of the foremost experts on fats and oils. Dr. Enig, through extensive research, has shown that the consumption of animal fat has actually decreased from 83% of total fat consumption to 53% in the North American diet over the last 80 years. In this same time, vegetable fat consumption has jumped from 17% to 47%.

It is Dr. Enig's belief that this rise in consumption of vegetable fat is correlated with the rise in cancer. But the vegetable fat that Dr. Enig and many other fatty acid researchers are most concerned with is the unnatural trans fats from hydrogenated and partially hydrogenated oils. Trans fat is found in commercially available baked goods like bread, crackers, chips, cookies, pies, and doughnuts.

Trans Fats

"Frankenstein fats" is one name for the artificially altered fats that are more often called **trans fats**. Trans fats include those fats found in fried foods, margarine, and most bakery products. Trans fats have been chemically transformed through heat and hydrogenation (the process of filling in vacancies on the carbon chain by adding hydrogen atoms). By adding hydrogen atoms and altering the structures of healthy essential fats, food scientists give these fats longer shelf lives. Good for business, bad for health. By hydrogenating these once-healthy, biologically active fats, we alter them in such a way that they become even more easily incorporated into our cellular membranes. This quirk in our biochemistry causes much confusion at the cellular level, leading to a leaking effect in our cellular membranes and ultimately causing chaos with many biochemical functions, including the closing down of our fat-burning machinery. Trans fats have also been shown to increase insulin, decrease testosterone, reduce energy metabolism, increase bad cholesterol, and inhibit immune function, just to name a few of the side effects.

Unsaturated Fats

An unsaturated fat is a dietary fat with one or more positions where there is a double bond (=) on its carbon (C) chain (meaning there are openings for hydrogen atoms). There are two general categories of unsaturated fat:
- a monounsaturated fat has one double bond between two carbon atoms;
- a polyunsaturated fat has two or more double bonds (=) between adjacent carbon atoms.

Saturated Fatty Acid
C-C-C-C-C-C-C-C-C-C-C-C-C-C-C-C-C-C
Monounsaturated Fatty Acid
C-C-C-C-C-C-C-C-C=C-C-C-C-C-C-C-C-C
Polyunsaturated Fatty Acid
C-C-C-C-C-C=C-C-C=C-C-C-C-C-C-C-C-C

It is the positioning and number of double bonds along the carbon chain that give the various fats their special roles. The more double bonds the carbon chain has, the more biologically active the dietary fat can be, and the more places it can go besides the fat cell.

Fat and Carbs: The Deadly Duo

Remember, from Chapter 2, that fat requires both high lipoprotein lipase (LPL) activity and high insulin levels in order to be stored within your 30 billion fat cells. In the absence of LPL and insulin, dietary fat will have a very hard time ending up in your fat cells. But when dietary fat is consumed with large enough amounts of high-glycemic carbohydrates (stimulating LPL and insulin levels), then most of the fat and additional sugars from the carbs eventually becomes stored body fat.

Foods such as ice cream or potato chips that contain a lot of fat along with sugars are excellent combinations if you want to increase your dress size in a hurry. The sugar in these foods (yes, even from the broken-down starch from the potato chips) boosts your insulin and LPL levels, and the fat from these foods gets shuttled into your eagerly waiting fat cells straightaway.

Monounsaturated fats (MUFA) are important to overall health, especially when the goals are low blood triglyceride, low LDL cholesterol, and low glucose levels. A high consumption of MUFA contributes to a lower incidence of cardiovascular disease and diabetes. MUFAs also act as antioxidants, reducing the free radicals produced by LDL cholesterol oxidation. Research on people with diabetes has shown that a diet high in MUFA can reduce blood levels of triglycerides by 19%, LDL cholesterol by 14%, and V(ery)LDL cholesterol by 22%. That's a sizable decrease considering that many lipid- and cholesterol-lowering drugs don't deliver these kinds of results, and carry with them serious side effects.

Oils rich in MUFAs include olive, canola, and high-oleic safflower oil. They're a great addition to our arsenal of fat-fighting weapons. Mediterranean diets are high in MUFAs because of the high amount of olive oil consumed. As a matter of fact, Mediterranean people consume up to 40% of their calories as fat and still have some of the lowest incidences of heart disease in the world today. Just remember: MUFAs are high-calorie dietary fats themselves, so when adding them to foods, take away other calories from harmful fats or high-glycemic carbohydrates.

Not Just Good Fats—They're Essential

Linoleic acid (LA), known as omega-6, and alpha-linolenic acid (ALA), known as omega-3, are classed as essential fatty acids (EFAs). These dietary fats are different from other fats because the body cannot manufacture them; they must be consumed. They are both polyunsaturated. Omega-6 has two double bonds between carbon pairs, and omega-3 has three.

These two fats are considered essential because they supply the building blocks of various structures within the body. These include the cell membranes that enclose every one of our 100 trillion cells and the raw ingredients in the structures of eyes, ears, the brain, sex glands, and adrenal glands. EFAs also regulate the traffic of substances in and out of our cells, keeping foreign molecules, viruses, yeasts, fungi, and bacteria outside of cells, and keeping cell proteins, enzymes, genetic material, and organelles (like the mitochondria where fat is burned) inside the cells. Because EFAs carry a slight negative charge, they repel each other, spreading out in all directions to carry oil-soluble toxins from deep within the body to the skin surface for elimination. EFAs also store electric charges that produce the bioelectric currents important for nerve, muscle, and cell membrane functions and the transmission of messages from the brain.

Fatheads

The next time someone calls you a fathead, take it as a compliment. According to clinical neuroscientist and co-author of *Bio-Age: 10 Steps to a Younger You*, Dr. Michael Schmidt, "Not many people realize that the brain is nearly 60% fat, but science has unlocked this mystery further to reveal that over 50 different conditions of the brain may be associated with fatty acid imbalance or insufficiency." Dr. Schmidt describes the extraordinary ways in which fatty acids can be used to heal a variety of brain-related conditions in his book *Brain-Building Nutrition: The Healing Power of Fats and Oils* (North Atlantic Books).

Without an adequate supply of these friendly fats, our fat-burning potential again comes to a halt. Fat can actually help burn fat? Yes! These essential fats work together to increase the overall amount of oxygen utilized by the cells to produce energy. The more oxygen we transport to our cells, the faster we burn body fat. EFAs increase the body's metabolic rate and also increase the insulin efficiency of the body. Therefore, by making the omega-6 and omega-3 fatty acids the main sources of dietary fats, we can greatly reduce our unwanted fat stores.

The Essentials on Essential Fatty Acids
EFAs can:
- help keep insulin functioning properly;
- regulate oxygen and energy transport;
- help to form red blood cells;
- keep hormone-producing glands active;
- help make joint lubricants.

The Messengers of Fat Burning
Omega-6s and omega-3s are also precursors to a biologically powerful group of hormone-like messengers called eicosanoids. Eicosanoids are not secreted by glands (like endocrine hormones), and they don't travel far distances to relay their messages. Instead, they are continuously produced (in minute quantities) in our cells, existing for less than a few seconds. They affect nearly every biochemical process in the body. The group of eicosanoids that is directly involved in fat metabolism is called **prostaglandins (PGs)**. The E series of PGs are the ones most important to fat tissue regulation:
- **PGE-1:** Derived from the fatty acid gamma-linoleic acid, PGE-1s are considered "good PGs." PGE-1 helps to burn fat by acting as a control mechanism, slowing insulin secretion and increasing glucose tolerance. Studies on people with diabetes confirm that they usually have low levels of PGE-1.
- **PGE-2:** Derived from the fatty acid arachidonic acid (AA), PGE-2s are considered "bad PGs" when they are in excess, due to their ability to oppose PGE-1.
- **PGE-3:** Derived from the fatty acid docosahexaenoic acid (DHA), PGE-3s are considered "good PGs." They act as a weaker version of PGE-1.

It is of the utmost importance to note that all prostaglandins are important regulators of our biochemistry. However, when we produce excess amounts of the PGE-2 series, things get a little out of whack. When in excess (as is typically the case among North Americans), PGE-2s can be viewed as bad guys due to the powerful inflammatory potential they possess. In reality, we need this prostaglandin for many vital functions. The problem arises when the system is out of balance, when there is too much activity in this family. An imbalance of this prostaglandin can also be detrimental to your fat-burning efforts.

PGE-1 and PGE-3 from omega-6s and omega-3s are especially important because they:
- regulate blood pressure, platelet stickiness, and kidney function;
- help transport cholesterol;

Controlling the Enzymes

As you can see from the fatty acid conversion chart, fats must go through many biochemical steps before becoming PGEs. You will also notice that there are two specific enzymes that help control this action. The first, D-6-D, controls the conversion of LA to GLA. But, according to Dr. Michael Schmidt, the activity of D-6-D can be blocked by many different factors, including aging, vitamin and mineral deficiencies, medications such as corticosteroids and non-steroidal anti-inflammatory drugs (NSAIDs), smoking, fasting or starvation, high insulin/blood glucose levels, and obesity, just to name a few.

Many people, due to the above-mentioned factors, may not be manufacturing enough of the D-6-D enzyme for PGE-1 production to occur. I recommend supplements in Chapter 12 that help bypass this enzymatic step, allowing for greater PGE-1 production.

The second enzyme, D-5-D, controls the conversion of ALA to EPA, as well as the conversion of DGLA to AA (PGE-2). Insulin is the primary activator of D-5-D, while glucagon is D-5-D's primary suppressor. You can also take supplements recommended in Chapter 12 to suppress this enzymatic step.

ESSENTIAL FAT CONVERSION CHART

OMEGA-6	OMEGA-3
Your Diet	

LA ◄ DELTA 6-DESATURASE ENZYME ► ALA

GLA

DGLA ➤ PG-1 SERIES (GOOD)

AA ◄ DELTA 6-DESATURASE ENZYME ► EPA ➤ DHA

PG-2 SERIES (BAD)   PG-3 SERIES (GOOD)

The conversions of the essential fatty
acids to the PG messengers.

- help generate electrical currents that make our hearts beat properly;
- decrease inflammation;
- help stabilize moods (by acting as an antidepressant);
- help your immune system fight infections;
- help prevent the development of allergies;
- improve insulin sensitivity;
- build docosahexaenoic acid (DHA), which is needed by the most active tissues—the brain, retina in the eyes, adrenal glands, and testes (PGE-3 is primarily responsible for this function).

FOOD SOURCES OF ESSENTIAL FATTY ACIDS

Your body's cells are made up of untold trillions of fatty acid molecules. The balance of these fatty acids within your trillions of cells is determined largely by your diet. When you consume a balanced proportion of omega-6 and omega-3 fatty acids, your cells become balanced in these fatty acids as well. But when you are deficient in fatty acids from the omega-3 family, your cell membranes in turn become deficient. When your body sends the necessary signals, the fatty acids that form the structure of your cell membranes are transformed into various prostaglandins such as those of the "E" series. The following is a list of the foods that contain the precursors of those PGEs.

PGE-Series	Fatty Acid	Fatty Acid Family	Food Sources
1	Linoleic	omega-6	Sunflower, safflower, sesame, and corn oils, or anything made with these food items
1	gamma-Linolenic	omega-6	Primrose, borage, and black currant seed oils
2	Arachidonic	omega-6	Animal meat, milk, eggs, squid, warm water fish
3	alpha-Linolenic	omega-3	Flax, canola, pumpkin, chia, walnut, brazil nut
3	EPA	omega-3	Cold-water fish, krill, algae (some)
3	DHA	omega-3	Cold-water fish, krill, algae (some)

The EFAs are not always benign. Overconsumption of omega-6 is linked to an increase in certain cancers and an increase in obesity. When it comes to the maintenance of optimum health and increased fat-burning potential, a partnership between the omega fats is the best medicine, with omega-3 being the dominant player. It is the omega-3s (fish oils) that stand out in stimulating fat-burning activity, due to the fact that they help suppress PGE-2 activity.

CLA: The Fat Wars Smart Bomb

As mentioned in Chapter 5, conjugated linoleic acid (CLA) is a natural polyunsaturated fat found primarily in beef and milk. CLA has been shown over the years to have many beneficial effects on our physiology, some of which include potent antioxidant activity, anti-carcinogenic properties, anti-catabolic properties (stopping muscle wasting), and powerful immune system-enhancing capabilities.

The benefits of this incredible fatty acid would most certainly require a separate book, but I have included it here based on two of the latest studies concerning fat loss and CLA in humans. The first study, presented in the *International Journal of Obesity* in August 2001, proved that CLA supplementation could reduce abdominal fat in men who were classified as abdominally obese. In this double-blind, placebo-controlled trial, 14 of the 25 participants who received CLA showed a significant decrease in their abdominal diameter after only four weeks of supplementation. The amazing thing was that none of these participants altered their eating or exercise habits during the study. The second study, presented in *The Journal of Nutrition* in December of 2000, followed 60 overweight or obese subjects over a 12-week period. Of the 47 people who completed the study, the average weight loss reported was 6 pounds. This study concluded that CLA is a promising agent in both the loss of body fat and the preservation of muscle mass.

The amazing thing about these two studies is that they were performed on people, not on animals. Animal research with CLA has continually shown remarkable results in all the areas presented in this section. It is nice to know that there are natural alternatives out there to help us in our continual war against our 30 billion fat cells.

Typically, in Western industrialized nations, human fat cells store more than 50% monounsaturated fatty acids, 30% to 40% saturated fatty acids, and 10% to 20% polyunsaturates. This is a reflection of the ratio of dietary fats we consume. Among the polyunsaturates in fat-cell triglycerides, less than 1% are from the omega-3 family. This means we're very much omega-3 deficient. Since 1850, omega-3 consumption has decreased to one-sixth its traditional (healthy) level, resulting in an omega-6 to omega-3 ratio of 20:1, with an optimum ratio being between 1:1 for the brain and 4:1 for the lean tissues. High levels of omega-6 EFAs as a whole suppress the uptake of omega-3s into tissues. By increasing the amount of omega-3 essential fatty acids in our diet with foods like flaxseed oil and cold-water fish (containing EPA and DHA), we'll be able to reintroduce this important class of nutrients into our cells.

FINDING FATS AND STORING THEM

The most common oils are extracted from seeds (canola, flax, safflower, sesame, sunflower), grains (corn, wheat germ), fruits (avocado, olive), beans (soy), and nuts (almond, coconut, palm kernel, peanuts, walnut). These are the fats that you can most easily add to your diet.

The molecules in saturated fats are shaped like a straight line and are easily stacked together in a solid mass. These dense fatty acids are very stable; they resist damage from air, light, and heat. Saturated fats are found in butter and coconut oil.

Monounsaturated fats (high in oleic fatty acids) are less stable than saturated fats but more stable than polyunsaturates. When refrigerated they become thick, but at room temperature they become thin again. They are a wise choice when using oil for cooking purposes, but they should never be placed on high heat. Monounsaturated-rich oils include olive and canola.

Polyunsaturated fats are the least stable. Safflower, sunflower, and corn oils are the most popular polyunsaturated oils and require careful handling to ensure freshness. The super-polyunsaturated oils are the most rare and are rich sources of essential fatty acids. They are also the least stable. They are found in cold-water fish and oils from flaxseed and, to a lesser extent, in canola and hempseed oil (omega-3s) and in omega-6 seeds such as black currant, borage, evening primrose, safflower, sunflower, corn, and flaxseed. Oils like cold-pressed flaxseed oil and others are very sensitive to high temperatures. These oils degrade very quickly and should be refrigerated (or frozen) and kept in a lightproof, tightly sealed container. (Flaxseed oil sold in health food stores is packaged in an opaque bottle—or should be—and is likely refrigerated.) Unrefined oils like sesame and peanut oils are also very active and should not be used for cooking—they should not be exposed to high temperatures. Add them to salad dressings or other non-heated foods for the best results.

HOW MUCH DIETARY FAT IS ENOUGH?

Just how much dietary fat should a person consume, and what is the ideal ratio of the various fatty acids for maximum fat burning and optimum health? Some people do better on more fats than others, but in general, it's the type of fat that's important for improving the metabolic rate and allowing muscle cells to function at their full fat-burning and carbo-hydrate-storing potential.

Limiting the trans fats, saturated fat, and even the omega-6 fatty acid linoleic acid is a good start. I recommend that approximately 30% of your calories come from dietary fats—mostly essential fats. In other words, cut down on the animal fats and processed vegetable fats and consume more fish and flax oils to balance out the ratios of fatty acids. Use the recommendations in Chapter 14 to calculate your own requirements for daily fat intake.

KEY TACTICS

1. Not all fats are bad for you.
2. Don't replace fat with carbohydrates in your diet.
3. EFAs not only keep us healthy—they help us burn fat!
4. Try to consume more fats from the omega-3 family (see fatty acid food sources in Figure 7-1).
5. For an added bonus you may want to give CLA a try.

8

Macro-Fuel Three:
Dietary Proteins

Dietary proteins play a key role in health and fitness, but I want to make it clear (again) that a balance of carbohydrates, dietary fats, and high-quality dietary proteins is the answer when it comes to overall success with fat loss. Many people never reach their fat-loss goals because of an all-or-nothing approach to their diets. Research has overwhelmingly confirmed that if we consume a proper balance of foods while lowering our overall consumption of high-glycemic, insulin-spiking carbs, we will burn fat. Notice that I've never mentioned eliminating carbs, as so many diets currently advocate. The problem with this approach, as you will see in the next chapter, is that you end up causing your body to crave them even more. Winning the Fat Wars is all about having the right balance at the right times (Part III has more on balance).

Most of the high-protein diets we see on the market are really low-carbohydrate diets in disguise. Carbohydrates (high-glycemic) can cause us to gain unwanted fat, but removing them altogether from the diet is not going to solve the problem. To turn the tide, many researchers now recommend scaling back on (but not eliminating) the carbs and increasing the dietary proteins. But why are dietary proteins so important?

The importance of dietary protein has been documented since ancient times. The originators of modern medicine, the ancient Greeks, first named dietary protein "protos," which means "to come first" or "of the first rank." Every day our bodies build and rebuild close to 300 billion cells with the raw materials found in dietary proteins. Carbohydrates can supply energy for building these body proteins, but they don't supply the actual raw building materials. Only protein and certain fats can do that.

The proteins we get from our foods are made up of amino acids; there are about 20 amino acids that are considered biologically important to human life. Eight of them are considered essential, because the body cannot produce them on its own and must obtain them from our diet. The other 12 amino acids can be synthesized in the liver from these original eight. Special digestive enzymes called proteases break them down into individual amino acids and combinations of amino acids called peptides (di-peptides, tri-peptides, etc.). They are the building blocks for our organs, muscle cells, transport proteins, and enzymes. Dietary proteins are absolutely essential for life and fat-burning success. Remember that protein is the substance that stimulates the fat-burning hormone glucagon and builds metabolically active muscle. This is one of the reasons why proper protein consumption (which I write about in Chapters 12 and 14) is at the core of the Fat Wars program and is crucial to your fat-burning success.

We're not only what we eat; we are also what our ancestors ate. And guess what? Our ancestors ate lots of dietary proteins. As Dr. Boyd Eaton has pointed out (see Chapter 2), our early diet consisted of at least 30% protein. Of course, the protein our ancestors ate was a little different from much of the protein we consume today. Early humans consumed protein from lean game meats that also contained the essential fatty acids that are often lacking in our diets today. Other research indicates that we were predominantly hunters and then gatherers, but our ancestors had the same genes we have today. Our early ancestors were in some ways much healthier than the carbohydrate-loving, grain-fed humans of the agricultural revolution. According to case studies of prehistoric populations, these hunter-gatherers were tall, lean, muscular, strong, had dense bones, very little tooth decay (if any), and experienced very little disease.

PROTEIN VS. CARBS

Protein helps elevate our resting metabolic rate throughout the day and night—yes, protein helps you burn more calories even while you sleep! Compared with a high-carbohydrate meal, the thermic (fat-burning) response from a high-protein meal can be 40% greater, and that's a lot of extra heat. This may be due to protein's ability to up-regulate thyroid hormones and uncoupling proteins (see Chapter 1). Research also shows that protein meals increase oxygen consumption by two to three times the rate that a high-carbohydrate meal does; this also indicates a much greater increase in the metabolic rate. When protein is consumed with every meal, it helps increase our level of alertness and concentration by stimulating the brain chemical called dopamine (see Figure 8-1). High-carbohydrate meals have the opposite effect, leaving us feeling dull and sleepy. If we don't get enough dietary protein from the foods we eat, we'll slow our metabolism down to a snail's pace.

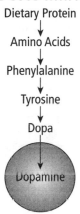

FEELING GOOD WITH PROTEIN

Dietary Protein
↓
Amino Acids
↓
Phenylalanine
↓
Tyrosine
↓
Dopa
↓
Dopamine

Figure 8-1: *The production process for dopamine, a feel-good chemical.*

Research also shows that a diet rich in proteins contributes to greater gains in muscle during resistance training than a high-carbohydrate diet does. High-protein meals are also more satisfying, filling us up better than a high-carbohydrate meal. High-protein (along with fat) meals decrease hunger, due to their ability to send satiation signals to the brain. The best sources of lean protein include chicken breast, turkey breast, fish, seafood, egg whites and whole eggs, cross-flow microfiltered whey, and lean meats like wild game and tenderloin cuts. Other good sources of protein include organic yogurt, organic cheese, organic cottage cheese, fermented soy (tofu, miso, or tempeh), and, of course, high-quality soy protein isolates.

Protein Supplements

Some newer dietary protein formulas that are very effective at curbing the appetite, building muscle, and burning fat are whey protein isolates that feature the AlphaPure trademark (recommendations are listed in Appendix I). One of the most important things you can do on the Fat Wars plan is to consume high-quality dietary protein with every single meal.

ALL DIETARY PROTEINS ARE NOT CREATED EQUAL

The actual value of the various dietary protein foods is measured in the Net Protein Utilization (NPU) Index, which reflects the biological value, expressed as a percentage of digestibility of a specific dietary protein. The biological value of dietary protein is the efficiency with which that protein deposits the proper proportions and amounts of the essential amino acids needed for anabolism (the building of body proteins). The important factor is not the amount of dietary protein consumed, but the amount of dietary protein that is available to the body after ingestion. And the better the quality of protein you consume, the faster the results will show up on your new physique.

Our bodies all have their own specific amino acid profile, and there is no one food that fits that profile exactly. Other than the dietary protein found in our own mother's milk (perfect protein), all other proteins are rated in the NPU against the next best thing: an egg. The only food that has a higher NPU than whole eggs is whey protein, but since whey protein is an engineered food of sorts, the egg remains the benchmark.

The Net Protein Utilization Index

Protein	BV (biological value)
High alpha whey isolate	(AlphaPure) 159
Cross-flow microfiltered whey isolates	110 to 159
Whey protein concentrate (lactalbumin)	104
Whole eggs	100
Cow's milk	91
Egg whites (egg albumin)	88
Fish	83
Beef (commercial)	80
Beef (non-commercial, venison, and elk)	80
Chicken (breast)	79
Turkey (breast)	79
Caseinate and milk protein isolates	77
Soy	74
Rice	59
Wheat	54
Seeds, nuts, legumes (beans), sea vegetables (spirulina and chlorella)	49

More About the Benefits of High-BV Proteins

If you consume only proteins that have a low biological value, then your body will have a much harder time utilizing the protein for structural (muscle, bone, organs, etc.) and functional (enzymes, neurotransmitters, hormones, etc.) products. Protein can also be broken down as an energy source by the body. The problem is that when protein is burned for energy, it creates metabolic waste products in the form of ammonia. These nitrogenous waste products can overload the kidneys and liver, causing potential problems in people susceptible to kidney and liver ailments. It is my opinion that the higher the quality of protein consumed, the more effectively that protein will be utilized for the important functions the body needs it for. Your body has plenty of fat and sugar to burn as fuel. You don't need to create extra waste for elimination by burning protein. It is better to consume smaller quantities of higher-quality proteins.

Plant-based dietary proteins, aside from non-GMO soy protein isolates, are very low on the list. A sizable portion of dietary proteins from vegetables are never absorbed because the fiber in these foods binds to the protein. (The only exception to low NPU ratings when it comes to vegetable proteins is some soy products.) Active vegans, who only consume 100% plant-based foods, have one heck of a time building and repairing muscle tissue. Many studies have shown that when an athlete's essential dietary protein supply comes exclusively from plant-based protein, that athlete begins to lose quality muscle and strength almost immediately. Many vegetable proteins are not only low in biological value (in terms of bioavailability), but also high in carbohydrates (particularly vegetables like beans, peas, and corn).

Most of the dietary proteins we eat should come from foods such as lean cuts of red meat (venison, tenderloin, lamb), white meats (skinless poultry and fish), some low-fat dairy products, and eggs. Many high-quality animal proteins these days (mainly beef, pork, chicken, and eggs) must be prepared carefully to avoid a host of infectious bacteria, including salmonella and E. coli. Animal protein can also be riddled with fat, so choose lean varieties. Fish remains an excellent source of amino acids and essential fatty acids. No matter what the source, be a smart consumer. Buy foods that are as fresh, organic, and free range as possible.

Additional dietary proteins should come from supplements of only the highest-quality protein powders containing whey isolates, soy isolates, or whey and soy blends. (See Chapter 12 and Appendix I for some recommendations.)

> ### *Protein and Testosterone Levels*
> In Chapter 3, I write about how easy it is for men (and women as well) to gain excess body fat as they age due to a decline in their testosterone levels. This loss of testosterone is invariably linked to the majority of testosterone becoming bound to the sex hormone transport protein SHBG. Once bound, testosterone is unable to exert its muscle-building, fat-burning effect on cells. It turns out that diet may actually have a big influence on the outcome of SHBG as we age, and protein just happens to be the star player. Research published in *The Journal of Clinical Endocrinology and Metabolism* in January 2000 showed that elderly men who had a low dietary protein intake experienced elevated SHBG levels and decreased testosterone bioactivity. This subsequent decrease in testosterone from low protein intake can result in a lot more than extra body fat. It can potentially result in declines in sexual function, muscle mass, and red cell mass and can contribute to the loss of bone density.

THE BETTER WHEY

Whey is a by-product of the cheese-making process. Whey was actually regarded as waste until scientists researched the profiles of its chemical protein structure and decided to try to extract that protein. Early whey protein products were referred to as whey concentrates. They contained as little as 30% to 40% dietary proteins and were filled instead with huge amounts of fat, lactose (milk sugar), and denatured (damaged) proteins.

> ### *Which Whey?*
> As mentioned in Chapter 5, some milk may negatively affect immune function. Due to a substance called the ABBOS epitope found in bovine albumin, milk can suppress the immune system. And since whey is a milk derivative, what stops it from containing the same potentially harmful substance? The answer is in the type of filtration used. Cross-flow membrane-filtered whey isolates (with cutoff values of 3–30 kiloDaltons) filter out all the harmful substances, including the ABBOS epitope. Therefore, this is the only type of whey isolate I recommend at the moment. Read your labels carefully.

These proteins are extremely anabolic and are able to increase protein synthesis faster and better than other dietary proteins. Their superior amino acid profile gives them the edge over other dietary proteins when it comes to their digestibility and incorporation into muscle tissue.

The most exciting thing about whey protein isolates is their ability to increase our immune response—particularly in the fight with cancer. The protein also aids in fat burning and muscle growth, works as an appetite suppressant, and can be used by those who are lactose intolerant.

The majority of the products available today come from newer processes—ion-exchange and cross-flow membrane extraction. They have a higher percentage of dietary proteins than their predecessors—high enough to merit the label "isolates."

The newest generation of whey isolates can contain more than 90% pure dietary proteins, with almost no dietary fats and minimal levels of lactose. They are also very expensive to produce. Due to the increased cost of the newer isolates, many manufacturers tend to mix the isolates with less expensive concentrates and still call them isolates. Only a very small percentage of companies use 100% isolates.

NON-GMO SOY ISOLATES

Soy protein isolates are a good alternative for vegetarians and, as mentioned in Chapter 4, "Her Fat," women going through menopause. The newer isolates closely meet human needs when it comes to the supply of valuable amino acids.

Soy isolates are high in the branched-chain amino acids (BCAAs), which are needed for muscle energy and growth, and are high in arginine, which is needed to stimulate anabolic hormones like human growth hormone (HGH). They're also high in the most abundant amino acid in muscle tissue, glutamine. Glutamine is another amino acid that drives anabolic metabolism.

Another effect of soy is its ability to lower bad cholesterol levels and increase good cholesterol levels. Soy protein does this so well, in fact, that as of October 26, 1999, the U.S. Food and Drug Administration approved the use of health claims regarding the role of soy protein in reducing heart disease. (It is normally against the law to make any health claim on a natural product without the approval of the U.S. F.D.A.)

The normal range for cholesterol in a healthy human being should be around 160 milligrams/deciliter of blood. The risk of cardiovascular disease starts to rise at cholesterol levels exceeding 200 milligrams/deciliter. Over 100 million North Americans have blood cholesterol levels over 200 milligrams/deciliter. That's almost half the North American population. More and more people are being measured with blood cholesterol levels over 240 milligrams/deciliter; that's almost a sure ticket to Heart Attack Alley.

As noted in the section on women and menopause, scientists have known for years that people in Asia have a much lower incidence of blood cholesterol and certain types of cancers. The relative absence of these diseases has been linked to the high consumption of plant foods, including soy. Soy protein increases glucagon levels, facilitates the fat-burning effect, and lowers cholesterol levels.

Even though there are many proposed benefits from consuming soy protein, there may also be possible hazards with excess consumption, according to newer scientific data from animals. Until we have a clearer understanding of whether the benefits outweigh the risks, I would advise a lower consumption of higher-quality protein isolates. I believe that fermented miso and tempeh do not pose any risks, but instead offer many advantages due to the fermenting process. For updates on soy, please visit *www.fatwars.com* on a regular basis.

HOW MUCH DIETARY PROTEIN?

According to the Recommended Dietary Allowances (RDA) set out in Canada and the U.S. for dietary proteins, we shouldn't be taking in any more than 0.8 gram of protein per kilogram of body weight. While this amount may be acceptable for people who never move, many researchers (including myself) believe that it is much too low for someone who wishes to gain muscle. There is actually a statement in the U.S. RDA Handbook that reads, "In view of the margin of safety in the RDA no increment is added for work or training." Apparently these experts are under the impression that nobody in the U.S. works, let alone works out.

This certainly does not mean that you should overconsume dietary proteins at any one sitting—too much protein in one meal can stress the liver and kidneys. The upper limit, depending on body size and activity level, seems to be 30 to 40 grams, or approximately 6 ounces of meat, at one sitting.

We're all biochemically different and therefore our dietary protein requirements are different. Just assume that the more active you are, the more dietary protein you will need to repair the body. Dr. Lee Coyne points out in his book *Fat Won't Make You Fat* that according to some of the most respected researchers in the field of nutrition, the RDAs for dietary proteins can be low by at least a factor of three. This assertion is further backed by research by Dr. Emanuel Cheraskin, formerly from the University of Alabama. After assessing the Cornell Medical Index Health Questionnaire filled out by 1,040 dentists and their spouses, Dr. Cheraskin found that those who consumed two to three times the RDA of dietary proteins had the fewest medical health problems.

Individual dietary protein intake and absorption is also affected by the way the proteins are prepared and the accessory nutrients that are available for the assimilation of the proteins. Dietary proteins require a full array of the B vitamins in order to be properly utilized and incorporated into body tissues.

One of the most effective ways to increase fat-burning potential is to increase anabolic metabolism (anabolism), the rebuild and repair process of the body. This is the rate at which we are able to turn over new cells and repair our bodies. Dietary proteins are the driving force behind anabolism, due to their ability to supply the nitrogen necessary for repair.

We are very complex structures of nearly 100 trillion cells. These cells are constantly regenerating, as our bodies replace our entire muscular system approximately every six months. Therefore, the nutrients we feed ourselves today will determine who and what we become tomorrow. The quality of dietary proteins we consume is of the highest priority. To help with protein requirements, I highly recommend protein shakes, so I've included sample recipes at the end of Chapter 11. These liquid protein meals may just give the fat-burning team the upper hand in the Fat Wars.

The importance of consuming only the highest-quality dietary protein can never be taken for granted. Since you are renewing the molecules of your structure every second of every day, you have to be accountable for what you put in your mouth, and what ultimately becomes part of your structure.

We recognize that we must all respect the ecosystem on earth so that we may breathe the air of the future. The human body is also an ecosystem, just as complex and beautiful as the world we live in, and it too demands respect. If we think twice about littering on this planet, why not think twice about littering in our own bodies?

I think the sports nutrition researcher Dr. Michael Colgan, Ph.D., said it best when he wrote, "Oh, the human system is ingenious at making do with inadequate building materials, patching, stitching and pinch-hitting, but it can't build premium tissue from garbage. A Twinkies-and-coffee diet produces a Twinkies-and-coffee body. For optimum performance you have to eat optimum protein to build optimum structure—period."

KEY TACTICS

1. Dietary protein is critical to building mass and burning fat.
2. Not all dietary proteins will work the same way in our bodies.
3. The higher the quality (BV) of dietary protein we consume, the more efficiently and healthfully our bodies use it to help us burn fat, build muscle, and regenerate our entire cellular composition.
4. Supplemental protein isolates (especially whey) are a great way to add high biologically valued proteins to the diet.

9

Constant Craving

Janice pulled her hand out of the cookie bag. Both were empty. Of course they were. It had taken her less than 10 minutes to scarf down the dozen or so White Chocolate Macadamia Nut Sensations. She felt a twinge of guilt as her tongue corralled a wayward crumb on her upper lip and swept it into her mouth.

So much for that diet. She'd lasted a whole seven days this time. Last time, the cravings got to her before the end of the third day. But then again, that wasn't totally her fault: Losing her job and having her car towed on the same day were more than any dieter should be expected to deal with. Besides, that tub of Triple Mocha Almond Fudge Surprise was not only much cheaper than a prescription for Prozac, it was—she rationalized—healthier for her in the long run. At least she'd been smart enough to buy the brand with 100% real cream; as a woman approaching her 40s, she knew she was at risk of developing osteoporosis and needed to build up her calcium intake.

This time, she wouldn't be so hard on herself. At least she was staying away from the cigarettes. So what if she put on a few pounds? She was saving her lungs from further damage. And winter clothing was so accommodating, really. If she wore enough layers on top of her skin, no one would ever notice the extra rolls forming beneath it.

This is how the Fat Wars are slowly but surely lost. Our own chemistry sets us up for defeat, and fat deposits grow throughout our bodies, despite our best intentions.

Janice is not alone when it comes to this seemingly never-ending desire to fulfill food cravings. The only problem is that we never seem to crave the right foods—the healthy ones. Most food cravings are fueled by the body's need for something it's lacking or by an addiction to the pleasure we feel from consuming these fat-inducing foods. That's right, from the moment you were old enough to eat on your own and your mother placed that first taste of sugary sin on your little tongue, your brain danced for joy and you were instantly hooked.

When I near the end of one of my many lectures on obesity and fat loss and it's question-and-answer time, the same question comes up time and again: "Why can't I stop eating carbs?" In this chapter, I will explain in detail why you may experience cravings that seem to overtake your senses, cravings that win control and push you further behind in the Fat Wars. I will take you through the latest scientific discoveries of why these carb cravings occur. Once you have a basic understanding of the whys, you will be able to construct the hows. As you read this chapter and start to understand why your body does what it does, I hope that you find yourself saying "Aha!"

CRAVING THAT HIGH!

Many carbohydrate-containing foods (like those White Chocolate Macadamia Nut Sensations Janice devoured) release a morphine-like chemical in the brain called beta-endorphin. Beta-endorphins produce a sense of well-being, reduce pain, ease emotional distress, increase self-esteem, and even create a sense of euphoria. From that first taste of sugar on your tongue, the pleasure center in your brain is awakened and beta-endorphins are immediately released.

The problem is that the feeling of satisfaction from these sugary foods begins to create a dependency (addiction) that eventually robs you of your health and overloads your fat cells through elevated insulin and fat storage enzyme (LPL) levels. Due to a mechanism in your brain's reward cascade system called priming, ingesting even small amounts of sugar on a regular basis can make you crave more. This priming mechanism is the reason why Janice, like you and me, can't be satisfied and stop at one cookie. That one measly cookie is like a drug you just can't get enough of, and it doesn't matter how full your tummy is, because your brain ain't listening.

Have you ever noticed that after a dinner party, no matter how stuffed you seem to be, as soon as dessert comes around you mysteriously seem to make enough room for it? This, once again, is the brain's way of saying, "Hey buddy, don't even try to deny me my high." And the problem just gets worse. Excess sugar creates excess beta-endorphin, which in turn causes the brain to start closing down some of its endorphin receptors (due to the surplus), eventually creating what I call endorphin defect. The endorphin defect is what causes the desire for the drug (sugar) to create the high all over again. Soon the only way to feel good is to continuously binge on junk food—the biggest drug of all.

Once the initial sugar high from beta-endorphin has died down somewhat, you start to feel a sense of calm and well-being. You experience this calming sensation after the high in part due to the slow-release action of another brain chemical called serotonin. Don't get excited yet, for you are about to discover how this chemical—like beta-endorphin—also creates a dependency, feeding yet again into the carbohydrate addiction cycle.

SINGING AGAIN WITH SEROTONIN

Serotonin, like beta-endorphin, is one of the body's neurotransmitters. Neurotransmitters are chemicals that transfer messages from one nerve cell to another, or from a nerve cell to a muscle cell. Think of our neurons as branches of a tree. As one branch extends, it sends a number of twigs off in various directions, reaching toward, but not connecting with, the twigs from another branch. The communication (telling the hand to grasp that cookie, for example) between these twigs happens through messages that are passed back and forth via the neurotransmitters. Studies have shown that different neurotransmitters affect different areas; serotonin has been shown to affect a wide variety of functions, including comprehension and memory, mood, temperature, aggression, and appetite.

Our bodies function on a feedback system: When a level of a component is too low, a message is sent out to increase it. If the amount of available serotonin is low for some reason, the body's feedback system springs into action to ask for a speedup in the production line. Our bodies look for the easiest and most direct way to bring the level of serotonin back up to what is necessary—and it just so happens that the consumption of carbohydrates is the way to boost serotonin. And we all know that junk food is filled with carbohydrates. As the high-carb foods raise our serotonin levels, we start to breathe a big sigh of relief. Unfortunately this feel-good sensation is quickly overshadowed as we pass that full-length mirror in the bedroom, the one that always seems to lie.

How Does Serotonin Work?

In the 1990s, Richard and Judith Wurtman, researchers from the Massachusetts Institute of Technology (MIT), began to suspect there was a link between low serotonin levels and eating disorders. Richard Wurtman had done studies in the 1970s with research student John Fernstrom that involved tryptophan, an amino acid (a building block of protein) and a precursor of serotonin. The body can't make serotonin without trypto-phan's help. They found that tryptophan rapidly entered the brains of rats that were fed a carbohydrate-rich diet (mostly starch and sugar), enabling the rapid production of serotonin. When they altered the rats' diet to include a protein component, the serotonin levels did not increase, nor was there increased activity in the systems that use serotonin.

Eventually they, and other researchers studying tryptophan, found that dietary proteins prevent tryptophan from entering the brain. In fact, tryptophan, which occurs in smaller amounts than all the other amino acids in protein, was actually bullied out of the way as it competed for pas-sage into the brain.

Where do carbohydrates come in? They don't usually contain trypto-phan; only protein-based foods (and some exceptions like bananas and pineapples) do. So how does eating carbohydrate-rich food increase the brain's levels of tryptophan, which increases the production of serotonin? When we eat carbohydrates, our digestive system breaks down the carbs into glucose, which can be transported in the bloodstream. Glucose in the blood stimulates the pancreas to release insulin, which escorts the glucose into the cells, where it becomes a source of energy. Amino acids are con-stantly surfing the bloodstream, so they get escorted into the cells as well. Remember how I said that tryptophan, in the presence of proteins, gets bul-lied out of position when it's trying to get into the brain? Well, as it's push-ing the other amino acids into the cells, the insulin is giving tryptophan a chance to get into the brain uncontested.

If it weren't for the fact that increased insulin interferes with fat burn-ing, we could call this situation a truce: The cells have their energy-producing glucose and amino acids for growth and repair, and the brain has its trypto-phan, from which it can produce serotonin on an as-needed basis.

Tryptophan and Serotonin
The average daily intake of tryptophan is around 1 or 2 grams. Only about 10% of this amount is actually used by the brain for serotonin synthesis (the creation of serotonin) due to the body's other needs for tryptophan (i.e., protein synthesis). When under excessive stress (and who isn't these days?), most tryptophan is converted into vita-min B_3 (niacin, niacinamide). Supplements containing B vitamins (especially B_6 and B_3) and perhaps even NAD (the active coenzyme form of B_3) may be helpful in directing more tryptophan toward sero-tonin synthesis. These B vitamins also help neurons manufacture more serotonin.

CRAVING CARBS

When you realize how often the body calls on its stores of serotonin—to help with sleep regulation, depression, anxiety, aggression, appetite, temperature regulation, pain sensation, and sexual behavior, to name a few—it's no wonder we can run low on serotonin at times. A low level of serotonin could be the result of either a depletion of the stores (through poor dietary habits and high stress, for example) or a decrease in the production (i.e., not enough tryptophan to produce serotonin).

One More for the Road

Ever wonder why some people can have a few drinks and party the night away, while others seem to want to sleep? The answer lies in what comes after the initial insulin rush from alcohol intake. Alcohol works like a refined carbohydrate, only it's much more concentrated (and much closer to fat in its caloric content of 7.5 calories/gram).

As you drink alcohol, it can attach to and activate your serotonin receptors. Some of us want to fall asleep soon after our first drink, due to the conversion of serotonin to the sleep hormone melatonin.

But in some individuals, just the opposite seems to happen. Because these people have used up most of their serotonin, when the alcohol binds to its receptor, it instead activates the uplifting neurochemical dopamine (discussed in Chapter 8). It's these people who respond to that first drink with a dopamine rush who can drink all night. Just like those cookies, one drink is never enough. The more alcohol these people drink, the lower their serotonin levels fall and the higher their dopamine levels climb. With empty serotonin tanks, these people become completely uninhibited due to a lack of serotonin impulse control. These are also the people who have the highest tendency to become alcoholics.

Any way you look at it, whether you fall asleep after a drink or ask the bartender to "hit you again," any excess alcohol will make you fat.

If we are eating to fight a low level of serotonin, why do we end up gaining weight? Regardless of whether we choose starches or sweets, it all gets reduced to glucose, initiating the insulin cycle. The problem is that it takes some time for serotonin to kick in, and we keep eating until it does. Besides, all of these carbohydrate-rich foods taste so good, we don't want to stop when we should.

What we don't know can make us fatter. While our bodies are waiting for serotonin to reestablish itself, we continue to scarf down fat-laden, high-carb foods. What we don't realize is that serotonin can take a lot longer to rise than we want it to, due to another unexpected messenger: galanin.

GALANIN

If the body is craving something, doesn't that mean it's needed? And shouldn't we give our body what it needs? Aha! Consider the difference between need and want. When we satisfy a carbohydrate craving with fat-laden foods, that enhanced euphoria (from beta-endorphin) followed by a sense of calmness (resulting from the increase in serotonin production) is quickly overshadowed by a feeling of lethargy. The more carbohydrate-rich, fat-laden food we eat, the more weight we gain and the more lethargic we feel. We are now officially part of the vicious carb circle—but now we're not only depressed again, we're fatter too! We're on our way to becoming overweight, depressed slugs.

What's going on? The answer, identified by Dr. Sara Leibowitz, a professor at Rockefeller University and a recognized world authority on neurochemicals, lies in the effect of a powerful neurochemical called galanin. This chemical is released once a certain amount of dietary fat has entered the body. Galanin competes with serotonin and quickly overpowers it, causing us to feel passive and tired and interfering with our ability to think. Oh, great! Now we're overweight, depressed, and *confused* slugs.

Galanin also creates a certain craving for fats. When you diet or skip meals (and you know who you are), free fatty acids trigger the release of galanin from the hypothalamus in your brain. Once galanin levels start to rise, you begin to crave fatty foods. Galanin is also triggered by reproductive hormones like estrogen (one of the reasons why women who experience PMS crave fatty foods), stress hormones like cortisol, and our old friend insulin.

Galanin levels peak in the evening, which is why we desire those fatty foods late at night. By creating the craving to eat at night, evolutionarily speaking, your body ensures extra fat storage (due to your lower metabolic rate) for that overnight "famine." We have a hard enough time losing fat as it is, especially when evolution is against our efforts from the start.

And just when you thought things couldn't possibly get any worse, in addition to creating fat-food cravings, galanin plays a key role in making sure that extra dietary fat gets deposited into your fat-cell accounts (as if you don't have a big enough balance already).

And the Beat Goes On . . .

Dr. Liebowitz has also shown through her research that high-carbohydrate diets are responsible for stimulating the production of a chemical similar to galanin called neuropeptide Y (NPY). NPY creates an ongoing dependency on still more carbohydrates. It's interesting to note that NPY is most active first thing in the morning (this explains why breakfast is the favorite meal of the day) in order to stimulate your need to eat high-carbohydrate foods that refill those glycogen containers that were emptied while you slept. Stress is another big stimulator of NPY (one more reason you want to pig out when you're stressed).

I believe that diets promoting one extreme or another (high carb/low protein, high protein/low carb, etc.) can cause imbalances in these neuro-chemicals, eventually leading to mixed signals that create an ever stronger desire to eat the very foods you were trying to avoid all along. It's through balance that we create the best environment for fat loss. Many of the cravings that have kept us fat probably started from an unbalanced diet.

SEROTONIN'S PARTNER—BETTER THAN A LULLABY

Do you remember Mom's remedy for insomnia? A cup of hot milk and a banana. How could Mom know that these tryptophan-rich foods played a part in our sleep cycle? She probably didn't. She was just doing what her mother did for her. But what they were both doing, in fact, is helping the body as it follows its own circadian rhythm—the natural sleep/wake cycle. Part of that cycle involves melatonin, which is produced when serotonin is depleted. That is, as our daily amount of serotonin is decreased, production of melatonin is increased. The mood-enhancing chemical (serotonin) makes way for the mood-lowering chemical (melatonin). Because both serotonin and melatonin rely on tryptophan as a precursor, consuming a diet that has a sufficient supply of tryptophan is wise.

Maintaining Tryptophan Levels Naturally

How do we keep ourselves supplied with tryptophan so that serotonin and melatonin can keep us ticking along? Tryptophan, the amino acid needed to manufacture serotonin, can be found in certain foods, including milk, bananas, pineapple, chicken, turkey, soy, whey protein, and yogurt. Soy happens to be one of the richest sources of tryptophan.

A double-blind, placebo-controlled study (the most respected of studies) published in the prestigious *American Journal of Clinical Nutrition* in June 2000 indicated that whey protein containing high alpha-lactalbumin levels could greatly increase plasma tryptophan levels in highly stressed individuals (AlphaPure is one example of such a whey protein—see Appendix I). The study also indicated a decrease in stress hormones and a reduced depressive state through the alteration of brain serotonin levels.

Melatonin Only Comes Out at Night

At nighttime, serotonin is converted into our body's sleep regulator, the hormone melatonin. This conversion is controlled by an enzyme called N-acetyl-transferase (NAT), which converts serotonin into N-acetyl-serotonin before becoming melatonin. The reason we don't produce melatonin during the daytime is that the activity of the NAT enzyme is slowed dramatically by daylight hours and intense light (electric or sun).

SYNTHESIS OF TRYPTOPHAN TO MELATONIN

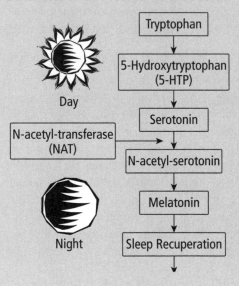

Since the U.S. Food and Drug Administration banned the sale of L-tryptophan as an amino acid supplement in 1989, the market has been forced to replace it with expensive prescription drugs. There are some natural alternatives as precursors, such as 5-hydroxy-tryptophan (or 5-HTP, as it is referred to in the health field), but trying the natural food approach first to top up your tryptophan tanks is always recommended. In Chapter 12, I also list alternative approaches to dealing with these cravings through various "crave-free" nutrients. These natural wonders have been shown in various studies to be a viable strategy for dealing with excessive cravings.

Hippocrates, the father of modern medicine, talked of the healing power of food. His motto was "Let food be your medicine, and medicine your food." In other words, when life got him down, he too probably would have reached for the ice cream, had it been available.

I have often witnessed people who, in desperation, decide to cut all carbohydrate-rich foods from their diet. Cutting out just the sweets and deep-fried snacks would work, but cutting out all carbohydrates will have a reverse effect. In fact, the fewer carbohydrates in your diet, the more your body craves them (to get the beta-endorphin and serotonin levels back up). A diet in which you eliminate carbohydrates almost completely may help you lose a few pounds at the beginning, but most of the weight you'll lose will be water, because each carb molecule is able to hold three or four molecules of water. Also, these diets will reduce your serotonin levels, so your body will send you on a carb binge when you go off the diet. (You always hate yourself when this happens—give yourself a break, and eat less-processed carbs in moderation.)

Eat, Drink, and Be Heavy

A new study published in *The American Journal of Clinical Nutrition* in 2001 found a direct correlation between the amount a person drinks and her dietary choices. The study, which looked at answers from a questionnaire submitted to approximately 73,000 French female schoolteachers, adjusted dietary intake by omitting alcohol-related calories. The respondents were split into two groups, based on their daily alcohol consumption. Heavy drinkers—defined as anyone who consumed over 2 1/2 alcoholic drinks per day—were shown to have consumed nearly 30% more calories from their daily food intake than non-drinkers. Heavy drinkers also had a tendency to consume more fatty foods, such as cheese, processed meats, and vegetable oil, along with more coffee, than the non-drinkers did. Alcohol is not only an appetite stimulant; it also causes depletion of your liver glycogen stores. As your liver glycogen declines, you start to crave carbohydrates—which accounts for the desire to eat a high-carb breakfast the morning after.

It's important to note that the moderate drinkers of this study had the best eating habits of all the participants, including the non-drinking group. The moral of this study is that if you decide to drink, do so only in moderation. Also, try to consume red wine (in moderation) as your alcohol of choice, to benefit from its antioxidant qualities.

What's more, your emotional state also plays a role here. Ever notice that when you're upset, your cravings for carbohydrates go through the roof? This is the body's way of telling you to pump up those neurochemicals to make you feel better, theoretically helping you deal with the emotional stress you're going through. The only problem is that you'll soon be under even more stress, due to the extra rolls of fat you've added from the extra carbohydrates. Nevertheless, oblivious to the future turmoil you are about to create, you reach for the carbohydrates again. Remember Janice at the beginning of this chapter? She used cookies and ice cream as quick, easy carbohydrates—just what her body ordered.

We all have our own addictions when it comes to satisfying our cravings. If the sweets aren't what you're looking for, you're probably guilty of going for the savory: chips and dip, perhaps, or a five-topping pizza? Yes, these foods do contain an abundant supply of carbohydrates that will eventually make their way into your body. The necessary biochemical conversions will take place, ultimately rewarding your pleasure centers by raising beta-endorphin and serotonin levels and supplying you with a great big sigh of relief. But the underlying problem with these foods is that they also deposit extra saturated fat into all your eager little fat cells, which are waiting like newly hatched chicks with their mouths wide open for their next meal.

These foods are manufactured solely for profit's sake, and without a care for your health. Don't think for one minute that the heads of these junk-food corporations go to bed each night thinking about how many people they've helped. They go to bed thinking about how much money they've made—at your expense, literally! The better these foods taste, the more you'll want to devour, and the fatter their wallets will become. And the more dietary fats these foods contain (especially animal fats—the worst kind for our bodies), the better they taste. When we are feeling down, we reach for these comfort foods, which satisfy us for the moment. But there's a better way. A new, healthier, slimmer, more energetic life. Aren't we worth it? Of course we are!

KEY TACTICS

1. Certain carbs (high-glycemic) create a chemical response in our brains to crave more carbs and fatty foods, creating a never-ending cycle.
2. The wrong carbs can also make us sleepy and lethargic.
3. Eating an unbalanced diet also triggers these chemical responses that cause us to crave more carbs and fatty foods.
4. Uncontrolled stress is another way to create insatiable cravings.
5. Unless we alter these neuro chemicals (i.e., serotonin) in our favor, we will never be ahead in the Fat Wars.

10

Starving

How many times have you been here and done this? One month has passed since the start of your latest diet, and you're finally ready to face the scale. For 30 days you've painstakingly cut the fat from every morsel of beef, peeled the skin off every breast of chicken, and opened your share of tuna cans. If someone were to ask how many calories are in a baked potato or a shrimp salad, you could snap back the answer with the speed of a winning contestant on Jeopardy. Cutting calories has left you hungry, tired, and feeling spacey at times, but you hope that this time it's all been worth it.

Stripped and ready to face the dial, you carefully shift your weight onto the scale. At first you cover your eyes. After all, fat is frightening. As you lower your hands from your eyes, you see that the dial reads a number you can actually live with. You've lost 12 pounds. You jump around the room, pumping the air and screaming "12 pounds!" But the question is: 12 pounds of what?

The real test comes next, as you nervously check the full-length mirror. This time things are going to be different. After all, the diet was a success and you've dropped 12 pounds to prove it. But as you gaze at the reflection, a stunned look quickly falls upon your face. There must be a mistake. The reflection you see staring back at you is not a leaner version of yourself, but instead a smaller fat person! Unless you're standing in the house of mirrors at your favorite amusement park, mirrors don't lie.

Don't think you're in the minority if you've failed at dieting. Contrary to those weight-loss ads you see in magazines and on television, 99% of all diets fail miserably. Diets fight our genetic makeup. They go against the way the body is designed to work. You may look like you're from the future, but the last time your body checked, you were still figuring out how to invent the wheel. Don't forget that the body has had centuries of training in the feast/famine cycle and it knows what to do to protect itself. It's not just that diets don't work. Most of them will leave you worse off than if you hadn't dieted at all. Once you finish the diet, not only do the lost pounds reappear, a few more are added for insurance against the next "famine." The more you lose, the more you seem to gain. What's wrong with this picture?

THE SCIENCE OF FAT RELEASE AND STORAGE

Remember our 30 billion fat cells? Not only can they expand, they can expand up to 1,000 times their regular size to store fuel as a reserve source of energy. These cells have specific processes (and enzymes) to trigger the storage of fat and its release. Science is now showing that obesity is usually caused by a dysfunction in one of these two systems—storage or release. Dieting plays a part here, by disrupting the balance of storage and release activity.

The two systems (as shown in Figure 10-1) are:

- **Lipolysis (the release of fat):** Lipolytic enzymes are enzymes that are responsible for the release of fat from our fat cells. Fat has to be released before it can travel to the fat-burning furnaces in our muscles. One of the most important of these enzymes is hormone-sensitive lipase. The more active this enzyme is, the easier it is for your body to get rid of its fat stores. Lipolytic enzymes are under the direct influence of the hormone glucagon.
- **Lipogenesis (the creation of fat):** Lipogenic enzymes are enzymes that are responsible for fat storage. One of the peskiest of these enzymes is lipoprotein lipase. The more active this enzyme is, the fatter you become. Lipogenic enzymes are under the direct influence of insulin. *Insulin stimulates the production of this enzyme so that it can store fat in the fat cells.*

When you over-restrict your calories, your body begins to produce more of the storage enzyme lipoprotein lipase. So by starving your body to lose weight, what you are really achieving, along with the loss of muscle tissue, is the production of more fat-storing enzymes, to give you even more of what you didn't want in the first place, fat!

Dr. Paul La Chance of Rutgers University analyzed 12 of the most popular diets in 1985 and found that all 12 relied on the reduction of calories to the point of serious nutrient deficiency. When we overrestrict our calories by following such diets, our bodies not only suffer from immediate deprivation, but also begin to produce more of the storage enzyme in order to pack away as much as possible, particularly after the period of severe calorie restriction is over. By starving ourselves to lose weight, we're actually setting ourselves up for a fat-storage marathon once the famine is over (especially when we lose muscle tissue).

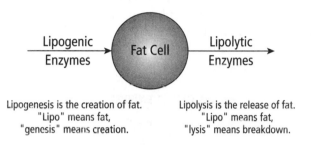

Figure 10-1: *Lipogenic enzymes encourage fat storage, and lipolytic enzymes encourage fat burning.*

Poll after poll shows that, at any given moment, over one-third of all women and one-quarter of all men are on the latest fad diet. Meanwhile, we know that other studies are showing that North Americans get fatter every year. Can you believe that we're spending nearly $40 billion a year on a diet industry that can't deliver results? If you opened a bank account and made weekly deposits, only to find out at the end of the year that you owed the bank money, would you assume it was your fault? Would you say to yourself, "I'll just have to save better next time," and open another account? Of course not, but that's exactly what you do when you go from one failed diet to another.

The Really Bad News About Diets
Low-calorie diets (in the absence of essential nutrients) not only deprive the body of valuable nutrients, but also cause a devastating loss of muscle tissue. "Who cares about muscle? I just want to lose fat!" you may say. Well, muscle is the prime site for burning fat. The more muscle we carry, the more fat we can burn for energy. Studies show that losing even 1 ounce of muscle lowers the body's ability to create energy and reduces our fat-burning capacity. When drastic weight loss occurs, this translates into a significant decrease in our resting metabolic rate—all because of this reduction in lean body mass (muscle). The reduced ability to burn fat sets us up for another round of the vicious cycle of losing fat and then regaining it, as our

new, post-diet body requires even fewer calories to function than it did before. See Figure 10-2 for an illustration.

Not convinced? Consider this:

- One pound of muscle can burn up to 50 calories a day.
- Fifty calories a day equals 350 calories a week, or 18,200 calories a year.
- There are 3,500 calories in 1 pound of fat. Therefore, a lost pound of muscle equals a loss of over 5 pounds of fat-burning capacity annually. If we don't reduce our calorie intake after the diet, those 5 pounds will likely find their way to some of our now-eager-to-store fat cells.

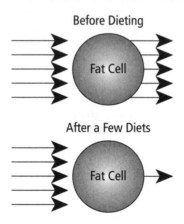

ARROWS DEPICT ENERGY RELEASE

Before Dieting

After a Few Diets

Figure 10-2: *Dieting can prime your system for fat storage.*

The message is clear: By losing valuable muscle tissue, we are turning down our metabolism, the main engine in the fat-burning process. Every time we diet, we lose more muscle, lower our metabolism, and prime our fat-storing enzymes. We're setting ourselves up for more fat gain, which is exactly what's happening.

Fat is burned within our muscle cells. Increasing the amount of muscle tissue, not putting all our energy into cutting calories, is what will ultimately increase the size and efficiency of the fat burners.

THE STRESS HORMONE CORTISOL

The culprit in muscle destruction is our hormonal systems. Our various hormones regulate many metabolic events in the body. Some of our hormones are *anabolic,* meaning they help to build body tissues. Testosterone (yes, even for women) and growth hormone come to mind. Other hormones can be considered *catabolic*, meaning that they stimulate a breakdown of body tissues. The most well-known catabolic hormone is cortisol, a hormone released by the adrenal glands when we are under stress. When we diet—subjecting ourselves to an artificial famine—our bodies consider themselves to be under stress, although cortisol production is also stimulated by traditional stressors—like when your car won't start on the day of the big meeting.

When the body recognizes this new stress, it releases a lot of adrenaline and cortisol. These two hormones are responsible for meeting the energy needs of the body in stressful times, and they truly want to help. This is the famous fight-or-flight response we've inherited from our ancestors, who really did have to fight or run for their lives to evade death. Our bodies have developed this incredibly quick response system to ensure the survival of the human race. By up-regulating our stress hormones, we can quickly break down sugars, dietary fats, and dietary proteins into their simplest components in order to supply energy and spare the fat stores. There's no telling how long the crisis will last, and stored energy in the form of fat is usually the last to go!

If there isn't a supply of new protein (amino acids) in the system, cortisol will have no other choice but to take it from our body tissues in a process called gluconeogenesis. Muscle tissue is the first to go. Cortisol steals nitrogen from the structural protein in our muscles. After removing the nitrogen, cortisol rapidly converts the protein to sugar for increased energy and maintenance of blood-sugar levels in the brain. This is long-term damage, and a major reason why we gain back weight after a diet. Cortisol eats the muscle that we use to burn fat. Here's an easy equation to remember: Excess stress equals excess cortisol, which oftentimes equals fat gain. (And we thought we gained weight during times of high stress because we chow down on so much comfort food. Well, that too.)

As we know, any loss of muscle is a victory for the fat side. Fat wins every time we lose even an ounce of muscle. To spare muscle, we've got to reduce the level of cortisol and/or raise our level of anabolic hormones. I've already mentioned that cortisol is increased during a reduced-calorie diet or fasting. The more calories you deprive yourself of, the more cortisol is produced. But dieting is not the only way to increase cortisol levels. They're also elevated during many other life stresses—illness, in-law visits, work-induced panic attacks, being caught in a traffic jam, losing a job, losing a loved one, or having too many bills to deal with. You're pumping out stress hormones daily, often with no let-up or release. And often you're stressed over anticipated events rather than actual ones. Any way you look at it,

stress is stress, whether it's real or imaginary. A famous quotation from
Mark Twain says it all: "I have been through some terrible things in my life,
some of which actually happened." In order to win the war on fat, you have
to change your perceptions, and learn to face many of the events in your
life with some degree of calm.

> ### Getting It Anywhere It Can
> Cortisol is produced along the same biochemical pathway as other
> hormones, including sex hormones. The body can only produce so
> many hormones, and if it's pumping out loads of cortisol, it won't have
> enough material to produce normal amounts of other hormones.
> Cortisol will always win out over the others to keep itself in abun-
> dance during times of stress. For instance, cortisol will compete with
> testosterone—ever wonder why you don't have a sex drive when
> you're stressed out, or why you lose muscle mass and strength?
> As I have repeated throughout *Fat Wars*, you can't win the
> war if you lose the very tissue that burns fat. With continuously
> high cortisol levels, your testosterone will be used up when it's
> needed for muscle-tissue synthesis. Cortisol competes with prog-
> esterone, which is one of the reasons why women have irregular
> menstrual periods when they are stressed out! Cortisol will also
> compete with dihydroepiandosterone (DHEA), which is also needed
> to burn fat. Remember the cortisol/DHEA balance from Chapter 4?
> When this balance favors cortisol over DHEA, your body really
> begins to break down.

The shock method of dieting away the fat just isn't going to work. The
body senses this stress and reacts accordingly. When you alter your dietary
patterns by going on a low-calorie, low-fat, low-protein, or low-carb diet,
the body picks up on it right away and sends out a stress response. No one
fools with nature! And as if that weren't enough of a problem, dieting also
decreases the production of your fat-burning enzymes and increases the
production of your fat-storing ones!

As I mentioned in the last chapter, stress also causes you to have an
insatiable appetite for high-sugar foods, due to the increase in the carbohydrate-craving neurotransmitter NPY and the decrease in serotonin. An
already compromised situation is further exacerbated. After the stress, your
brain continues to send out feed-me signals to refuel the reserves that have
been emptied.

Insulin and Cortisol: The Tag Team

Almost every one of your body's 100 trillion-plus cells can burn either fat or glucose as fuel, but the brain (under non-fasting conditions) relies heavily on available glucose for energy. Your brain uses almost one-half of your body's total blood sugar (approximately 100 grams) per day. Unlike the other organs of the body, which require insulin to pump glucose into their interiors, your brain is able to absorb glucose independent of insulin, which gives it first priority over the other cells of the body, unless insulin levels are kept chronically high through consumption of insulin-spiking carbs all day long. In that case, the breads, pastas, and other refined foods that you're eating will spike your insulin and in turn may keep the sugar from entering your brain.

As you saw in Chapter 2, glucagon is responsible for raising low blood-sugar levels, thus allowing sugar to remain accessible to the brain. If glucagon can't do its job properly because its actions are being blocked by high levels of circulating insulin, then the brain must look at alternative routes of accessibility. Your brain will do whatever it must to ensure its primary fuel supply, even if it means the other cells of the body go without. The tissues of the body are made insulin resistant for the sake of the brain. This is where cortisol enters the picture. Cortisol, in addition to cannibalizing existing body structures to make glucose, lessens the amount of glucose used by other cells, thus causing insulin resistance.

Even though cortisol may be trying to help the brain in one way by raising blood sugar and cutting off the supply to the other structures, excess cortisol is a bad thing. Along with cortisol's effects on degrading our metabolic engines (muscle), it has been shown to affect the memory-producing center of the brain by destroying hippocampal neurons. (The hippocampus is a horseshoe-shaped region of the brain, located in the temporal lobe. It has a role in emotions, memory, and sexuality.)

TAKE TWO PILLS AND CALL ME WHEN YOU'RE SKINNY!

Scientists have mapped out the key hunger and satiety (fullness) signals that the body uses to modulate appetite and have discovered that they are regulated by a control center in the brain called the adipostat. The adipostat is like the thermostat that regulates the heat in a house. It can signal that we are hungry ("I'm famished!") or it can signal that we are satisfied ("I can't eat another bite!"). Dieting puts these signals into turmoil by increasing the stress response (cortisol), with the hunger response coming out as the victor. When we diet, the adipostat's hunger mechanisms are set on high and our metabolic rate is lowered to conserve energy in case of a famine.

Glycomacropeptides (GMPs)

Glycomacropeptides (GMPs) are low-molecular-weight protein peptides that exert an antibacterial and antimicrobial effect on our biochemistry. But it is their amazing ability to stimulate a hormone that can control our hunger responses that has obesity researchers most excited.

GMPs are powerful stimulators of a hormone called cholecystokinin (CCK), which plays many essential roles in our gastrointestinal system. CCK stimulates the release of enzymes from the pancreas and increases gall bladder contraction and bowel motility. CCK can also regulate our food intake by sending satiation signals to the brain, making it a potential diet aid. In animal studies, a rise in CCK is always followed by a large reduction in food intake. In human studies, whey protein glycomacropeptides are shown to increase CCK production by 415% within 20 minutes after ingestion.

On another note, GMPs may also have the ability to prevent indigestion and heartburn. In rat studies, GMPs were able to decrease acid secretion in the stomach by 53%. One can only wonder what other effects from GMPs will be discovered in the future.

Not all whey protein isolate, contain GMPs. Ion-exchange whey protein contains trace amounts or no glycomacropeptide fractions at all. The AlphaPure high-alpha whey protein contains at least 20% of this important peptide fraction (see Appendix I). So if you're looking for a natural way to reduce excess hunger pangs, look for higher-quality cross-flow microfiltered whey proteins that list the amounts of GMPs they contain on their labels.

These hunger signals are so important that major pharmaceutical companies have spent millions of dollars to develop drugs that will control them. Eight new drugs approved by the U.S. F.D.A. work by altering a person's metabolism, signaling the brain to increase the satiety (feeling of fullness) response. The ninth and newest weight-loss drug, called Xenical (Orlistat), does not stifle hunger but does prevent the absorption of dietary fat from the gastrointestinal tract (kind of like the natural shellfish extract chitosan).

Obesity drugs were never designed for use as a quick fix when it comes to fat loss. Dr. Samuel Klein, M.D., professor of medicine and director of the Center for Human Nutrition at Washington University's School of Medicine, stated in a June 1999 editorial in *The American Journal of*

Clinical Nutrition that "drug therapy may be most useful for maintaining rather than achieving weight loss." But still, many over-fat and obese people look to the quickest fix possible, even if side effects come with the deal.

There are no quick fixes when it comes to successful long-term fat loss. Our bodies love fat. They love to store fat, and they hate to give it up. They're like Fat Scrooges. That's why fat loss is such a battle. Developing an understanding of how we can win the war on fat is our best hope, and I will show you how in the following chapters.

KEY TACTICS

1. Diets do not work! They disrupt the normal human cycles of self-preservation and the body subtly resists them.
2. Diets not only don't deliver results, they harm the body over time, depriving it of key nutrients and breaking down muscle tissue, creating a lowered ability to burn calories.
3. Dieting primes our systems for fat storage by increasing lipogenic (fat storing) enzymes.
4. Balance is the key to long-term success on any transformation program, and don't forget to reduce your stress levels.

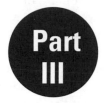

Part III

Let the Change Begin!

"The greatest discovery of any generation is that human beings can alter their lives by altering their attitudes."
—Albert Schweitzer

Now it's time to start thinking about how to use your new knowledge to make the necessary changes in your life—the changes that will take you, one step at a time, toward your own victory in the Fat Wars. In my experience, if you heed the following advice, not only will the fat melt off, it will stay off. Parts I and II of this book have put you in the Know Zone by explaining how your body functions and why you may be over-fat right now. These sections have also given you a new understanding of why all those previous diets put you on the losing side of the battlefield in the Fat Wars. You should now be well equipped with the knowledge of what needs to be done to move beyond your constant battles against your 30 billion fat cells.

Now that you have mastered the Know Zone, it's time to move into the Do Zone. You've always had the power to make the right changes, but the difference now is that you know how to make them in a way that makes sense for you.

It's time to choose your battle strategy. Your strategy will not be the same as anyone else's, because you are fighting your own Fat War. In the past, you may have been a yo-yo dieter or even a binge eater. Many people have to conquer their fear of failure due to many failed attempts at fat loss. Rest assured that the Fat Wars program is unlike any other weight-loss program you've ever undertaken. Gone are the diets that brought you down, creating a depressed and irritable state, driving you back, over and over again, to the waiting arms of your favorite comfort foods.

This time, you can lose a considerable amount of body fat and gain useful muscle, strength, health, and control at the same time. By the end of Part III, you will be able to take your newfound battle skills and design your own fat-loss plan. The following chapters will guide you through the eating and exercise principles, and suggest supplements that can help speed your progress. I will map out the first 45 days, then give you advice on how to proceed to keep seeing results for the rest of your life.

As you read about how to design your own eating and activity plan, resolve to start it today. *Fat Wars* is not another diet book; it is a life plan. The synergistic technologies and strategies presented in *Fat Wars* will help you end the war with your body and move on to peace with a leaner, healthier one. Is fat loss easy? You already know the answer to that question—with evolution up against you from the start, of course not. After all, if fat loss were that easy, you wouldn't be having such a tough time figuring out its secrets, and you certainly wouldn't be reading *Fat Wars*.

Is it possible to live a life without bags of excess fat weighing you down and robbing you of your health and vitality every second of every day? You bet it is! Permanent fat loss is about to become easier than you ever thought possible. And if you are willing to make the commitment for the next 45 days, then by the end of your 45-Day Transformation Period, you will not only look like a new person, you will be a new one. So what do you say? Let's stop procrastinating and get started!

11

The Fat Wars
Eating Principles

***Fat Wars* is not intended** to be another diet book. I don't want to get into various dieting strategies for weight loss; instead, I want to focus my attention on natural ways to increase the body's ability to burn fat. While this aspect is key, I wouldn't be doing justice to you if I didn't discuss daily optimum calorie consumption. The combination of effective eating strategies along with the activities and nutritional supplements that I recommend in this book is what makes this plan so effective.

In order to increase muscle and your energy levels and to burn fat, you need the proper fuel for your body. Energy comes from fuel and fuel comes from food. This means you must eat, and you must eat regularly (no, I'm not crazy). The key is to supply your body with the right fuel at the right intervals. Think of the example of the old clunker and the sports car. A person with a slow metabolism is like the old clunker. The old clunker won't give its owner much performance; it just sputters along— happy not to break down along the way. The clunker often guzzles gas and doesn't use it efficiently as it chugs along. The person with a slow metabolism usually doesn't use his or her fuel efficiently either—most of it gets stored as a fuel reserve (body fat). In contrast, a person with sufficient muscle and a fast metabolism is like the sports car. The sports car will give its owner all the performance he or she needs, but it requires the right kind of fuel at the right time to keep performing optimally.

Since metabolism is the speed at which the body processes food into energy, metabolism is the defining factor of body composition. Here's where diets also fail: When you limit the amount of food you take in, your metabolism adjusts by slowing down. The reverse is also true. If you supply your body with sufficient food, your metabolism will adjust by speeding up. (However, "sufficient" does not mean gluttony.)

Snack Your Way to Greater Fat Loss

When people set out to lose fat, often the first thing they do is go on a diet. When dieters deprive themselves of nutrition and calories, the first things they cut are snacks, not realizing that the right snacks can play a useful role in winning the war on fat. Dieters who eliminate snacks usually end up eating more at their main meals, quickly packing on the fat. When people hear the word "snack," they immediately think of junk food, instead of natural food. But there are healthy snacks that can fill the void between meals when blood sugar dips. Dips in blood sugar, if left unattended, lead to excess calorie consumption at the main meals and possibly to binge eating to satisfy cravings. When I refer to snacking in the Fat Wars plan, as you will see, I'm really referring to eating smaller meals more often.

In order to burn fat the Fat Wars way, you should never let more than three-and-a-half waking hours go by without eating something. If you go without food for more than four hours, blood-sugar levels tend to dip and the body starts to prepare for fat storage by switching into its prehistoric starvation-protection mode. In my own and other researchers' experiences, the ideal length of time between meals is from two-and-a-half to three-and-half hours. This way your body never turns on its storage switch.

When I say a meal, I'm not referring to major, calorie-dense meals. I am referring to meals that are between 300 and 500 (no more) calories. This means that they must be calorie-sparse yet nutrient-dense. This calorie range at each meal seems to be optimum for maximum fat-burning potential. Any more than the 500-calorie allotment and the body will be more apt to store the excess as fat (especially if you end up consuming more calories than you can burn). Of course, I can't overstate the importance of a balance of the macronutrients (carbohydrates, dietary fats, and dietary proteins) at each meal. The last meal is something of an exception, in that it should contain as fibrous and low-glycemic a carbohydrate as possible—a good serving of lettuce is a great choice. Consuming this sort of carb with your final meal is imperative for overall success on the Fat Wars plan because it allows you to burn more fat while you sleep (due to the depletion of glycogen reserves).

Meal Frequency

I have always recommended more than the usual three solid meals per day to my clients. We were all led to believe that breakfast-lunch-and-dinner is the way we should be eating. Those three solid meals we used to consume in the old days were actually quite nutritious. Not only that, we also performed enough physical activities to burn off most of the fat. Well, things have changed.

Consuming five smaller, nutrient-dense meals per day instead of three big ones will help you win the Fat Wars, as long as the meals are metabolically and hormonally balanced. When you eat this way, your body never has to plan for a famine by switching on its fat-storage genes. Sugar levels stay balanced, so the body never has to create stress and degrade muscle tissue to bring the sugar levels up again. And your body stays in a positive anabolic balance so that it can burn fat as its main energy source. See Figure 11-1.

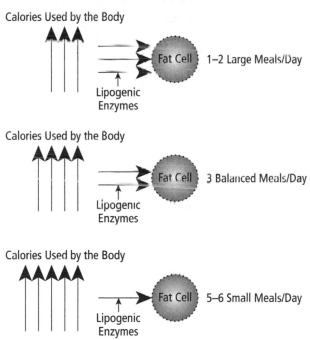

ARROWS DEPICT ENERGY RELEASE

Figure 11-1: *Showing the advantage of eating smaller meals more often.*

One thing I've learned along the way with various clients is that most people have a hard time with compliance. We are very busy people these days. Whether you are a businessperson, an athlete, or a homemaker, preparing (let alone consuming) five meals per day can be very arduous. This is one of the reasons I recommend two liquid protein meals per day. As you will see, they are not only lightning-fast to prepare, but also (if prepared properly) nutrient-dense, yet calorie-sparse. This means that you would be consuming three solid, balanced meals per day—just like you probably do now—and adding two liquid meals as well.

Macronutrient Profile

I've done my best to stay away from recommending any of the myriad diets on the market today. Fat Wars is not a diet plan; it is designed as a life plan in which you can benefit from your new knowledge of how the body stores and burns fat. However, there's so much confusion in the diet industry about the calorie allotment of foods and the macronutrient profile of these foods that I've decided to clear the air.

For best results in applying the Fat Wars eating principles, I have found that the carbohydrate content, the dietary fat content, and the dietary protein content should all be in ratios that are optimal for fat-fighting effect, all the while stifling your cravings for the wrong foods. I have analyzed the profiles of the leading diets, and the one that I believe works best for the majority of the population is the 40-30-30 plan.

The 40-30-30 plan refers to the breakdown of the various macronutrients. Carbohydrates make up 40% of each meal, dietary fat is no more than 30% of each meal, and dietary protein comes in at 30% also. This way of eating was first popularized by Dr. Barry Sears, author of *The Zone*, which takes into account that eating is indeed a hormonal event and that we are only as good as our last meal, hormonally speaking. I agree with many of *The Zone's* principles but I do not agree with all the recommended food choices. Many similar plans on the market seem only to be concerned with hormonal control of insulin and glucagon (which is important for fat burning), but not as concerned with food choices that take into account overall health and longevity.

I mentioned in Chapter 2 the many disorders in addition to fat gain that the hormone insulin can cause. In order for an eating strategy to be successful for lifelong fat loss, it must take into consideration the effect that foods have on insulin. This is one of the reasons why I do not believe in a high-carbohydrate diet; our prehistoric ancestors (with whom we share 99.99% of our genes) consumed a balance of foods closer to the 40-30-30 way of eating. I recommend following this eating profile as closely as possible at each meal (except for the last meal of the day).

- **40% carbohydrate sources.** Minimize items such as starches and sugars from processed foods, white breads, pasta, and polished rice. Maximize low-glycemic foods such as certain vegetables, legumes, fruits, and some whole grains. Carbs provide fuel in the form of glucose (blood sugar) for both brain and muscle activity and help to control food cravings by enhancing serotonin levels.

- **30% dietary fat sources.** Minimize items such as butter, cheese, beef fat, lard, trans fats (found in processed foods such as pastries and doughnuts), margarine, French fries, and potato chips. Maximize fats from the omega-3 and omega-6 family, such as flaxseed oil, fish oils, olive oil, nuts, and avocados. Fats assist in the balance of blood sugar, provide raw materials for hormones, create fuel for long-term energy, and strengthen cell walls and mucous membranes. They also control satiation and allow the body to burn fat instead of make fat.
- **30% dietary protein sources.** Good sources include lean meat, chicken breast, fish, low-fat cottage cheese, soy, and whey. Dietary proteins help to stabilize blood sugar; promote cell growth and repair; assist hormone production; assist in enzyme production (digestive and metabolic), neurotransmitter production, cell metabolism, and body fluid balancing; and maintain the immune system. Don't forget that protein also stimulates glucagon production, leading to more fat being burned as an energy source.

In order to keep muscle tissue at optimum levels and assist the body in maintaining all of its other functions, the body must remain in a constant anabolic (growth-promoting) environment. Following these general principles when eating will ensure maximum anabolic effects, which will ensure maximum fat-burning potential. Figures 11-2 and 11-3 go through what happens when you eat the typical way and when you follow the Fat Wars plan.

EATING A TYPICAL HIGH-GLYCEMIC CARBOHYDRATE MEAL

You consume a high-glycemic carbohydrate meal.

As the sugars from the carbohydrate are released in your mouth, your tongue initiates endorphins (feel-good hormones) within minutes, producing a feeling of satisfaction, calm, and euphoria.

Glucose floods the bloodstream, travels (without the aid of insulin) through the blood/brain barrier, and you start to feel good.

Figure 11-2: *A poor diet yields poor results.* (Continued on next page.)

The pancreas releases insulin to deal with the excess sugar.

Insulin forces blood glucose down and stores excess blood sugar short term as glycogen in the muscles and liver.

The insulin-stimulated enzyme lipoprotein lipase converts any leftover glucose that has not been stored as glycogen or used for immediate energy into body fat (at least 40%).

Since blood-sugar levels are now low, you begin to feel irritable, depressed, and sluggish.

Your body begins to beg for another high-glycemic carbohydrate meal (or snack) to raise blood-sugar levels again, and the whole scenario starts over.

Figure 11-2: *A poor diet yields poor results.*

EATING THE FAT WARS WAY

You consume a proper balance of low-glycemic carbohydrates, good fats, and high-quality protein.

As sugars are released in your mouth, your tongue initiates endorphins, making you feel good. Blood levels of all the amino acids rise, including tryptophan.

Glucose, along with the amino acids, trickle into the bloodstream, passing through the blood/brain barrier, and you start to feel good.

The pancreas releases a regulated amount of insulin that escorts the glucose and amino acids into the muscle for repair and into the liver to supply energy for the brain.

Figure 11-3: *A good diet yields . . . no surprise, positive results!* (Continued on next page.)

The pancreas releases the hormone glucagon.

The glucagon-stimulated, hormone-sensitive enzyme lipase initiates the fat release mechanisms so that fat can be used as a primary fuel.

Since blood-sugar levels are now stabilized and you are burning fat as a primary fuel source, you begin to feel energetic, with a sense of well-being.

As your hormonal environment is properly balanced and you continue to burn fat for energy, you feel full and satisfied for three to four hours.

Figure 11-3: *A good diet yields . . . no surprise, positive results!*

CIRCADIAN EATING RHYTHMS

Circadian rhythms are the natural daily patterns of the various processes within our bodies. They are often in tune with the cycle of daylight and darkness. For example, the levels of human growth hormone (HGH) rise and fall in a fairly standard rhythmic pattern throughout the day and night, peaking when we're in our deepest phases of sleep. The male hormone testosterone is another example, it peaks in the morning and then slowly falls. Almost every biochemical function that occurs naturally has a corresponding circadian response. Hunger and eating cycles are no different.

Because you produce most of your energy in the day and begin to shut down at night, your decisions about when and what to eat should take into account this metabolic cycle. Why would you eat little or nothing for breakfast when you want to produce a great deal of energy in the morning? For that matter, why would you eat an enormous dinner when you are going to be fast asleep not too soon after? Poorly timed eating is where many of us lose a battle in the Fat Wars.

In order to take advantage of our natural rhythm of fueling and activity, we must realize that most of our fat will be burned during the waking hours when our metabolism is at its highest. Therefore, we should synchronize our eating to the rate at which our metabolism is able to utilize the fuel sources. Metabolism is at its highest in the daytime, with the morning being the best time to start burning fat.

Too many people attack this in a backward fashion. Many people think that if they skip breakfast, then they will have one less meal in their system to make them fat. Wrong! This is like starting a long car trip without any fuel in the tank. The body needs fuel in the morning to rev up its engine. (Working out first thing in the morning after the night's fast will rev your engine up even more. The morning is the best time to get those fat-burning hormones working because they can keep working for hours afterwards.)

People usually make the mistake of eating not only the wrong amounts of food, but also the wrong kinds of foods throughout the day. Think of a typical breakfast of sugar-laden cereal or fried goodies, which are all high in high-glycemic carbs and the wrong types of dietary fats. These foods, as we have noted, will shut off your fat-burning machinery for hours, and your fat-burning success is only as good as your last meal (hormonally speaking). The same people who either skip breakfast or eat an unhealthy one come home from work famished and usually sit down to their biggest meal of the day, which again consists of the wrong foods. Soon afterwards, it's bedtime, usually still with a full tummy, and guess what? Their bodies now have ample time to store fat until the wee hours of the morning.

Here are some suggestions for eating the Fat Wars way:

- The largest meals should be consumed in the morning, with the size of your meals declining throughout the day. Alternatively, eat equally balanced meals throughout the day. No one meal should be higher than 500 calories. I've found that it's always best to leave the stomach less full rather than too full. That way, the stomach has an easier time mixing its digestive juices, allowing for a more efficient digestion of the food.

- Since high insulin works in opposition to human growth hormone (HGH), the evening meal should have little or no carbohydrate source, other than low-glycemic vegetables. Eating the right vegetables will allow low-glycemic carbs into the system without disturbing the HGH cycle. Eating a last meal that doesn't spike your insulin is the key to burning fat all night long.

- Try to eat at least every three-and-a-half hours for optimum fat burning.

- At least two of the meals should consist of Fat Wars shakes, which contain quality dietary protein and fruit from the berry family (preferably blueberries) or the melon family. Ten shake recipes are included in this chapter, along with their macronutrient profiles. If you work out in the morning, one of the shakes should be consumed immediately after working out.

- Stick to foods that are on the low side of the Fat Wars Glycemic Index. This is very important. If you combine eating low-glycemic carbs with the rest of the Fat Wars plan, success can be expected.
- Because dietary proteins are the key metabolic enhancer of the macronutrients, consuming dietary proteins at every meal is also very important.
- One to two tablespoons of organic flaxseed oil should be consumed each day to supply your body with essential fatty acids to help burn body fat (try adding the oil to your shakes).

FAT WARS SHAKES

A powerful blender could be one of the best investments you ever make. By using whole fruits as your base and adding water for the appropriate consistency, you will be adding great-tasting phytonutrition to your diet the way nature intended it to be delivered.

A Word About Juicing

These days, everyone seems to be into juicing. We're bombarded by infomercials on how healthy juicing is for us. I'm not here to rain on your parade, or anyone else's for that matter, but the fact is that juicing isn't for everyone. Throughout this book, I have mentioned the myriad problems associated with high blood-sugar levels and their effects on insulin—the hormone with the most impact on our metabolism. This is why I am emphatic about the importance of reducing your consumption of high-glycemic or fast-releasing carbohydrates and sticking to more complex, slow-releasing ones, such as those found in fresh organic fruits and vegetables.

As I noted in Chapter 6, all carbohydrates eventually break down into sugar in the body. It doesn't matter whether you consume 1/4 cup of pure sugar or eat a baked potato. They both are the same amount of sugar to your body (eventually), and your body will take the appropriate steps to bring the sugar level back into balance, which means producing insulin, which means fat can't be burned. The body works best with a very small margin of blood sugar, and anything that upsets this balance spells trouble for the entire system. Of course in the example above, insulin levels would not increase as fast with a baked potato as they would with table sugar. Refer to the Fat Wars Glycemic Index as often as needed.

When you consume foods like fruit juice, especially without the natural skin and pulp of the fruit, you are supplying concentrated sugars to your already overworked system. The human body isn't meant to consume fruit that's been stripped of its skin and pulp. The skin is also usually where most of those important phytochemicals are found.

Fruit juice—whether store-bought or made at home—also increases the calorie value of the shakes without providing other valuable nutrients. Remember, you're trying not to go over the 500-calorie mark with each meal, including the Fat Wars shakes. The only time I would consider pure juice is with the Fat Wars shake that you consume *after* your workout. This is the one time that your body shouldn't have any problems processing the sugars into stored glycogen instead of stored fat.

Please don't get me wrong. I'm not trying to stop you from drinking fruit juice. Instead, I want you to be aware that fruit juice, in enough quantity and like most everything else, can also become fat in your body, thanks to the body's miraculous biochemistry. What I suggest is that, instead of using pure juice, try blended whole fruit.

By using naturally flavored shakes supplemented with dietary protein formulas, you will be able to cut down on your overall calorie consumption without sacrificing nutrient intake. If you need fruit juice to give your shakes a sweeter taste, try diluting the juice—use half juice and half water—and remember to use your discretion when choosing your beverages. One final note concerning the Fat Wars shakes: Remember that nothing takes the place of good, clean water.

A Word About "Natural" Sweeteners

Some manufacturers try to gain leverage in the market by using sweeteners that supposedly are as natural as they come, such as fructose, commonly found in fruit sugar. Don't be fooled! Fructose found in fruit is actually good for us; when you take it out of its natural environment (fruit) and use it as a sweetener, it begins to cause trouble. In 1998, Dr. Levi and Dr. Werman did a study using rats fed a fructose-rich diet. The results showed that these rats had higher levels of damaged hemoglobin (which interferes with red blood cells' ability to carry oxygen) and higher levels of lipid peroxidation (which increases oxidation of fatty membranes by free radicals) than the rats fed a sucrose- or glucose-rich diet.

Our most prominent connective protein, collagen, can be damaged through high fructose consumption. Other findings suggest that long-term fructose consumption may actually accelerate the aging cycle.

Fructose is hidden in many processed foods and beverages in the form of high-fructose corn syrup. Many nutritionists recommend fructose as an alternative to sucrose for individuals with diabetes or reactive hypoglycemia, since fructose does not cause drastic fluctuations in blood-sugar levels. Life is too precious to take chances, especially when there are "true" natural alternatives to take advantage of. It's best to support the companies that make the extra effort in trying to bring you, the consumer, the healthiest of ingredients.

Shake Recipes

When adding any of the various ingredients that I suggest, such as fruit or yogurt, try to use organic products whenever you can. The nutrient content, as well as the lack of contaminants, will be well worth the extra cost. The following is a list of 10 of my most popular protein shakes. All of them are under 500 calories, and therefore can be readily burned by your body without surplus calories heading for your fat cells. They are also balanced to contain all three of the macronutrients for maximum satiety (fullness) potential. Try each of them, and come up with your own shakes too. These liquid meals will supply your body with the high-octane fuel it needs to build muscle and burn fat. Enjoy!

- **Shake Tip #1:** When mixing specialized dietary protein isolates, add the protein isolates to the shake as the last ingredient to avoid harming the delicate protein bonds. Blend for only a few seconds on low speed (just long enough to mix them in). Doing so will ensure that the high-quality dietary protein reaches your body undamaged by the heat created from the blending process.
- **Shake Tip #2:** The macronutrient values listed with each shake give the approximate value of each nutrient. These recipes are not intended to be followed to the letter. Use your own discretion when making these shakes. Based on your individual dietary protein needs, which you will calculate in Chapter 14, you may need to increase or decrease the amounts of protein that you add. However, I have tried my best to give you a pretty fair guideline to follow.
- **Shake Tip #3:** Even though it's already liquid, always chew your shake for a few moments before swallowing. Doing so ensures maximum digestion, since digestion starts in the mouth, through saliva. After all, food can't help us lose fat if it isn't digested and absorbed effectively.

The base for all the Fat Wars shakes contains:
- 1 ounce unflavored or natural vanilla–flavored protein isolate powder (whey, soy, or mixed)
- 1 tablespoon flaxseed oil
- 1 cup water

Combine these ingredients in a shaker cup. Shake until smooth. The following table contains 10 Fat Wars shakes. Note that "EFA" stands for essential fatty acids. (See Chapter 7 for more information on EFAs.)

Shake	Add To Base	Approximate Values
Fat Wars Blues	1 cup blueberries 1/2 cup blueberry low- fat yogurt 1/2 cup water	Calories: 445 Protein: 30 g Carbs: 43 g EFAs: 14 g
Black and Blue	1/2 cup blackberries 1/2 cup blueberries 1/2 cup water	Calories: 450 Protein: 30 g Carbs: 25 g EFAs: 14g
Boys Are Back in Town	1 cup boysenberries 1/2 cup water	Calories: 316 Protein: 25 g Carbs: 25 g EFAs: 14 g
Cranapple Sour	1 medium apple 1 cup cranberries 1/2 cup water	Calories: 378 Protein: 30 g Carbs: 41 g EFAs: 14 g
Tangy Tease	1 cup fresh-squeezed grapefruit juice 1 cup gooseberries	Calories: 480 Protein: 30 g Carbs: 45 g EFAs: 14 g
Green Berets	1/2 cup fresh-squeezed orange juice 1 banana 2 kiwis	Calories: 485 Protein: 30 g Carbs: 68 g EFAs: 14 g

Strawberries
  Battlefields
	1 cup strawberries
	1/2 cup low-fat
	  strawberry yogurt
	1/2 cup water
		Calories: 415 g
		Protein: 30 g
		Carbs: 38 g
		EFAs: 14 g

Crazy Feelin'	1 cup pineapple 1 cup watermelon 1/2 cup water	Calories: 430 g Protein: 30 g Carbs: 47 g EFAs: 14 g
Mellow Melon	1 cup fresh-squeezed orange juice 1 cup diced cantaloupe	Calories: 435 Protein: 30 g Carbs: 45 g EFAs: 14 g
Energy Edge	1/2 cup fresh-squeezed orange juice 1 cup pineapple 1 cup blueberries	Calories: 489 Protein: 30 g Carbs: 58 g EFAs: 14 g

For Athletes or Intensive Exercisers
If you are an athlete or a high-intensity exerciser and you are using one of these shakes as a post-workout shake, I would highly recommend carrying pure protein (about 20 grams) in a shaker cup with you to the gym or your event. After training, add water to the protein and then mix and drink immediately. Approximately 30 minutes later, mix your regular protein shake with fresh fruit, organic flaxseed oil, and organic honey (1–2 tablespoons). Following this suggestion allows for maximum recuperation due to the immediate rush of amino acids from the protein without reducing HGH and testosterone levels. The second shake allows for repair as well as glycogen replenishment. I have used this with many athletes with great success.

YOUR FAT WARS BLOOD TYPE

Everyone seems to be into blood typing these days. It's a concept that was popularized by naturopathic researcher and physician Peter J. D'Adamo, the author of *Eat Right for Your Type*. The main premise behind the blood-type dietary concept concerns how the four main human blood types evolved and how these blood types affect individual metabolism. If you are a follower of this unique concept, you can still apply the Fat Wars eating strategies to your individual blood type. Here is a very brief rundown of each blood type.

- **Blood Type O:** The oldest blood type, evolved around 40,000 B.C.
- **Blood Type A:** Emerged as humans became agriculturists, anywhere from 25,000 to 15,000 B.C.
- **Blood Type B:** Emerged in the Himalayas anywhere from 15,000 to 10,000 B.C., and became more widespread with the later expansion of nomadic people over the Eurasian plains.
- **Blood Type AB:** The newest of the blood types, evolved around 10 centuries ago.

Since there is strong evidence that the various blood types represent metabolic, and therefore dietary, differences, due to the types of foods these ancestors ate, there is a distinct possibility that many of us could have inherited differences in digestion and absorption capabilities for various foods. If you are a believer in this concept and want to design your Fat Wars food plan around your blood type, here are the dietary recommendations for each blood type. Simply alter your Fat Wars plan to include your personal blood type food recommendations, all the while sticking as close as possible to the 40-30-30 profile.

Blood Type Main Food Choices

- **Blood Type O:** Consume lean protein foods, including meat, fish, and poultry. Avoid all dairy products, grains, and legumes.
- **Blood Type A:** Consume mostly vegetarian-based proteins, along with fish. Avoid red meat and dairy products.
- **Blood Type B:** Consume all protein groups. Avoid corn, lentils, peanuts, and sesame seeds.
- **Blood Type AB:** Consume mainly vegetarian proteins, including fish, yogurt, and cottage cheese. Avoid red meats and most dairy products, with the exception of the ones listed.

Note: Through numerous dealings with clients and colleagues, I've come to believe that advanced whey protein isolates made using the cross-flow microfiltration process can be utilized, even by milk-sensitive blood types such as O, A, and AB. This is due to the superior filtration process that removes lactose (milk sugar), casein (the main milk protein), and all other impurities from the whey.

KEY TACTICS

1. Eat five times each day to avoid triggering "famine" responses in your body, which cause deep sugar cravings and ultimately a build-up of fat.
2. A 40-30-30 eating profile is recommended, paying attention to the quality, quantity, and kind of carbs, fats, and proteins you consume.
3. Hunger and eating cycles follow predictable patterns in a typical day. Understanding them helps you develop a personal plan that fights fat build-up.

12

Top 10 Supplements
for Fat Loss

I hear it all the time: "Because I eat right, I don't need supplements." Nothing could be further from the truth. Nutrient-poor diets contribute to disease, low energy levels, and obesity. If you think poor nutrition is limited to developing countries, think again. Recent research conducted by the U.S. Department of Agriculture shows that the nutrient value in crops is significantly less than it was just 20 years ago and is getting worse by the decade.

New studies point to the myriad benefits of consuming additional nutrients. Although these studies are not conclusive in the eyes of the government, they are in the eyes of the people who have experienced the benefits of supplements. One of these benefits may be living longer with your health intact; I call this "health longevity."

In the last 20 years or so, the total number of chronically disabled North Americans has dropped significantly (by almost 50%). So what does this have to do with nutritional supplements? Well, maybe nothing. But if you review the dietary supplement sales in this time period, you may be as convinced as I am. In 1982, North Americans purchased over two billion dollars' worth of these supplements. By 1999, the number had jumped to 15.4 billion. That's a seven-fold increase. One of the main reasons we are experiencing an increase in healthy longevity is a decreased disease risk and an increase in average life expectancy. Could this improvement in health have anything to do with the substantial increase in supplement consumption? I, for one, am not going to wait around for long-term human studies that may never come.

> ### *Making Our Foods Healthier*
> Our failing food system can be revived—if we start to develop crops
> that extract more nutrients from the soil (and increase the nutrients
> found in the soil), increase the diversity of food crops, reduce the
> loss of nutrients that occur with current harvesting and manufac-
> turing practices, and change the selection of the foods we consume
> to allow for better nutrient absorption. Until then, it's time to get
> realistic about our diets and admit that often what we eat does more
> harm than good. I often say that many people are starving to death
> on a full stomach. They're digging their graves with their forks.

My advice, and the advice of many other researchers and professionals in the health field, is to take out cellular insurance by consuming specific supplements. The supplements that I recommend in this chapter
contain one or a variety of special nutrients that aid the body's ability to
neutralize toxins and carcinogens, fight free-radical damage, control excessive cravings, produce energy, and increase your metabolism to burn fat. A
smart supplement regimen will go a long way to helping you win the Fat
Wars. It's one of your major weapons, along with healthy foods, proper
exercise, and sufficient rest.

While no magic pills are out there, a number of effective nutrients can
help to increase your ability to burn fat—as long as other lifestyle factors,
like diet and exercise, are taken into consideration. I have carefully
researched the top supplements available today pertaining to weight loss,
and have listed the top 10 supplements that could serve as your allies in the
Fat Wars.

Supplements are reinforcements that help to put the odds in your
favor. While each fat-burning nutrient or combination of nutrients that I
mention in this chapter helps to improve (directly or indirectly) your fat-
burning systems, some can do a lot more than fight fat. The goal is to prevent your muscle cells from becoming sluggish and weak—weighed down
with saturated and trans fats, low in fat-burning enzymes and transport
proteins, and unreceptive to insulin. By taking the various fat-burning
nutrients that are recommended, you'll immediately turn the tide of your
personal Fat War in your favor. Specific product recommendations are
listed in Appendix I; what follows is a general discussion of the nutrients
and what they can do.

Does taking supplements mean that you can slack off on your diet,
not exercise, get little sleep, and still lose lots of fat? NO! Remember: There

are no magic pills. The right combination of all the necessary lifestyle factors is what guarantees a victory.

For People with Diabetes

Some of the nutrients in this chapter can improve the sensitivity of muscle cells to insulin. When the cells are more receptive to insulin, less insulin is needed to entice the insulin receptors into allowing glucose into their structures and out of the bloodstream. As your body produces less insulin, it produces more fat-burning enzymes, transport proteins, and healthy mitochondria (those little fat-burning engines). And if you are an over-fat person with Type 2 diabetes, you may find these nutrients very helpful in controlling your blood-sugar level, reducing your percentage of damaged, oxygen-carrying hemoglobin, and melting the fat. What a bonus!

However, a word of caution is in order. These cell-sensitizing agents can have a profound influence on lowering blood-sugar levels. If you are on medications such as insulin, Metformin, and/or sulfonylureas that lower blood sugar, using some of the nutrients listed may require you to reduce your medications in order to avoid hypoglycemia (low blood sugar). I have seen this happen frequently. If you have concerns about your blood sugar or if you have diabetes, consult your physician or diabetes educator before using these nutrients.

1. PROTEIN ISOLATES

The key to long-term fat loss is building healthy muscle cells that can accept fat and burn it up. All the key structures that accomplish fat burning are protein based, so ingesting sufficient amounts of protein at regular intervals during the day is critical. Fortunately, we can incorporate high-quality proteins into our diet quickly and easily. Dietary protein powder isolates can be mixed with just about anything to create a high-powered protein shake in minutes.

These protein isolates enable our bodies to rebuild and repair themselves (the process of anabolism) faster than ever before. Anabolism creates the optimum environment for proper muscle recovery, not only from workouts, but also from the everyday stresses of life. The more effective your body becomes at anabolism, the better equipped it will be to burn off unwanted fat.

The two top protein isolates available today are high-alpha cross-flow microfiltered whey and non-GMO soy.

Whey Protein Isolates

Whey protein, a by-product of cheese production that was formerly considered useless, is the highest-quality protein known to science. It also can be fat- and lactose-free. The many advantages that whey protein isolates have over other protein sources include:

- They exit the stomach faster than other protein sources, providing a substantial, rapid rise in blood amino acids. The result is enhanced anabolism.
- Lactose-free forms of whey enable people with lactose intolerance to benefit from whey's superior amino acid profile.
- They help to stimulate the release of the hormone glucagon, which stimulates fat burning.
- They stimulate the liver's release of special polypeptides called somatomedins, which control the rate of muscle growth.
- In clinical settings, whey isolates have been shown to increase the immune response by up to 500%, due to their high levels of the amino acid L-cysteine.
- Whey contains a small protein compound called glycomacropeptide (GMP), which decreases appetite levels by stimulating the release of an appetite-suppressing hormone called cholecystokinin (CCK). In recent studies, GMPs from whey protein were shown to raise CCK by a whopping 415%.

A number of different types of whey protein are on the market. Becoming a smart consumer is important. Quality whey isolates are extremely expensive to produce, so many companies blend their formulas with cheaper concentrates. If you're buying whey protein and want the GMPs, remember that cross-flow membrane-extracted whey is the only version that contains them (unless they are re-added to a formula).

Also look for a high fraction of alpha-lactalbumin whey. This low molecular-weight fraction is quickly absorbed into the system, allowing for better repair of the muscle tissue. High-alpha whey isolates have also been shown to increase one of our most important antioxidants—glutathione— more effectively than anything else. The higher the glutathione levels in the body, the healthier we are.

Note: As I recommend in Chapter 8, try to look for whey isolates that use the cross-flow microfiltered (through membranes) process with cutoff values of 3–30 kiloDaltons (phone the manufacturer if you are uncertain). By using these types of isolates, you can reap the rewards of quality whey protein without subjecting yourself to any possible hazards associated with whey that is not produced using this stringent processing method.

Beta-lactoglobulin

Supplements that are high in beta-lactoglobulin (Betapure, for example), also have their advantages, especially where athletes are concerned. Along with alpha-lactalbumins, beta-lactoglobulins are the other major element in whey isolates. They contain unsurpassed levels of branched-chain amino acids that are needed to produce energy in working muscles and to build and repair new tissues. But the higher the quantity of naturally occurring alpha-lactalbumin, the easier it is for the body to absorb and utilize the protein.

Soy Protein Isolates

Soy proteins were the first protein powders available as a supplement. However, previous extraction technology did not allow soy to be isolated effectively, destroying most of the beneficial isoflavones (plant chemicals) in soy. Newer isolation methods allow for an incredible protein isolate that retains an abundance of these tiny, powerful heart-disease and cancer fighters and fat-loss helpers.

Soy isolates also contain some of nature's highest quantities of branched-chain amino acids (BCAAs) and glutamine. BCAAs and glutamine make up the majority of amino acids in muscle tissue and provide fuel for muscle function and repair. Here are some of the advantages of soy protein isolates:

- They contain the special phytochemicals/isoflavones genestein and diadzein, which have a variety of potent effects on the body, including inhibiting certain types of cancer.
- They have been shown to increase bone density in postmenopausal women by increasing estrogen levels and reducing the formation of osteoclasts (the cells that degrade bone).
- They can inhibit cardiovascular disease by reducing platelet aggregation and the oxidation of low-density lipoproteins.
- They can also act as a natural diuretic, because the isoflavones increase kidney function.
- They may help menopausal women lose fat by acting as estrogen supporters (see Chapter 4, "Her Fat").

Bio-DIM Absorbable Diindolylmethane

Nutrition researchers have always told us to eat our fruits and veg-etables. Fruits and vegetables contain phytonutrients (plant chem-icals) that are capable of exerting powerful, positive effects on our bodies. Even the simple soybean, tomato, or blueberry is a miracle of complexity. Scientists presently estimate that there are 30,000 to 50,000 bioenergetic phytonutrients in plants. Only 1,000 of these have been isolated so far, and only about 100 of these disease-preventing plant compounds have been analyzed and tested. One of those exciting phytonutrients was discovered in cruciferous vegetables; it is called diindolylmethane, or DIM for short. Bio-DIM is one supplement I highly recommend.

As mentioned in Chapter 4, "Her Fat," taking absorbable DIM is wise for most women to consider these days. But DIM is far from being only a woman's supplement. After all, men also produce both good and bad estrogens. Besides its benefits for healthy estrogen metabolism, Bio-DIM acts directly to create a more active cellular metabolism. Diindolylmethane uniquely activates protein kinase A, sensitizing fat cells to fat-burning hormonal signals for more efficient release of stored fat. In this way, Bio-DIM works together with com-plementary phytonutrients that are found in cayenne pepper, green tea, and grapefruit to support and facilitate weight loss. These com-bined phytonutrients represent a breakthrough in safe metabolic sup-port for the more active utilization and consumption of body fat during a weight-loss program.

The quality of the soy protein you choose can make all the differ-ence—the key is its active isoflavone content. Many mass-produced soy products, including tofu, lose vast amounts of their isoflavones during processing.

The traditional Japanese process of fermenting soy foods retains the foods' isoflavone content and even enhances the activity of the iso-flavones. When it comes to soy protein powders, only water-extracted soy protein isolate retains its natural isoflavone advantage. It is also very important to choose a non–genetically modified soy isolate. According to the U.S. Department of Agriculture, over 57% of soy products currently on the market are from genetically modified soy. If the packaging doesn't say otherwise, the isolate is likely from a genetically altered source. Please read the labels!

Other Benefits of Protein Isolates

Both whey and soy have unique qualities that assist you in attaining the physique you've always wanted. However, I highly recommend whey over soy when it comes to bioavailability and muscle-repair functions. You can take either one of these proteins alone, or combine them if you wish (a combined version of the two is listed in Appendix I). One of the benefits of consuming high-quality whey or soy protein isolates or a mix of the two is that you are guaranteed the exact amount of protein you need, without the added fat and carbohydrates—a definite bonus for any fat-loss program. Using protein supplements is the best way to fine-tune your dieting strategy. Together, the right kind of soy and whey isolates can offer an effective insurance policy against the breakdown (the catabolic processes) of the body.

2. ESSENTIAL FATTY ACIDS (EFAs)

As I wrote in Chapter 7, when it comes to the optimum functioning of your fat-burning machinery, it takes fat to burn fat. Feeding the body the wrong types of fats makes the cells dysfunctional (and lousy fat burners). You need to supply your body with friendly fat allies that you cannot make on your own. The right amount of these essential fats keeps the cells happy and helps them burn more fat. Those essential fats are omega-6 and omega-3, which are found in an optimum regular diet, but can also be taken in supplement form.

Omega-6 (linoleic acid) can be found in polyunsaturated safflower, sunflower, cottonseed, and corn oils, and is also present in high amounts in foods such as walnuts, wheat germ, and soybeans. Of the approximately 50 essential nutrients, omega-6 has the highest daily requirement—around 3% to 6% of your total calories per day (about 1 tablespoon). Remember that omega-6, with the help of the D-6-D enzyme, converts into gamma linolenic acid (GLA), which is a very powerful friend in the Fat Wars.

GLA can also be taken in a pre-formed source found in the oils of evening primrose, borage, and black currant seeds. Research seems to support the addition of either evening primrose or borage oils to your diet. Their pre-formed gamma linolenic acid (GLA) content ensures that your body has enough of this important fatty acid and also bypasses the D-5-D enzymatic step, allowing for proper PGE-1 synthesis.

Omega-3 (alpha-linolenic acid) can be found in large amounts in flaxseed oil and meal, perilla oil, and in lesser amounts in canola oil and hemp seed oil. Omega-3, like omega-6, has the ability to be transformed into closely related friendly fats such as eicosapentaenoic acid (EPA) and docosahexaenoic acid (DHA). Research has shown that omega-3 fatty acids help to improve brain function. (DHA is an essential fatty acid for the growth and functional development of the brain in infants.) Omega-3 fats are also able to help you lose body fat. One of the omega-3 fatty acids (EPA) lowers blood levels of triglycerides by increasing the transport of fatty acids into the cells for fat burning (thermogenesis).

Large quantities of omega-3 fats can be found pre-formed in wild cold-water fish such as Atlantic cod, Pacific halibut, sole, menhaden, mackerel, rockfish, salmon, and tuna. Farm-raised fish do not contain enough of these pre-formed omega-3s, likely because their diet is devoid of omega-3s.

By taking high-quality fish oil supplements that contain sufficient quantities of EPA, you can further help your body produce the good prostaglandins (hormonal messengers). High-EPA fish oils help to suppress the enzyme D-5-D, which is responsible for the end product of AA (the bad PGE-2). Insulin is the primary activator of D-5-D, while glucagon is D-5-D's primary suppressor.

Marine oils are very reactive and must be protected from heat, sunlight, and oxygen. EFAs are required in gram amounts daily and are highly perishable, deteriorating rapidly when exposed to air, light, heat, and metals.

If you choose to supplement your diet with extra EFAs, I recommend that you take 1 tablespoon of cold-pressed organic flaxseed oil with your Fat Wars shakes every day. In addition, take 1–2 capsules of molecularly distilled (i.e., no PCBs or mercury toxicity) cold-water (Norwegian or North Atlantic) fish oil with each meal. (Some research points to the enhanced benefits of enteric-coated fish oils for absorption purposes.)

CLA: A Fat That Helps Burn Fat?

One promising fatty acid is **conjugated linoleic acid** (CLA), which has been shown to reduce fat and increase muscle in animals. CLA seems to work by increasing the basal metabolic rate so that people trying to lose excessive fat can actually increase their caloric intake and still lose fat. It has also been shown to reduce the inflammatory prostaglandin PGE-2 by suppressing arachidonic acid.

CLA has also received attention as a potent antioxidant and cancer preventive. Even small concentrations of CLA in cells is enough to produce significant cancer (i.e., breast and prostate) protection, and this effect is independent of the other fatty acids. In addition to these benefits, CLA has also been found to be useful at burning body fat and increasing muscle mass. Researchers believe that CLA embeds itself in cell walls and helps to regulate the flow of nutrients into the cell and the flow of by-products out of the cell. In this way, CLA becomes a potent weapon for making cells more active, which, in turn, makes them more efficient fat burners. The recommended dosage is 1000 milligrams two to four times daily.

3. CRAVING FORMULAS (THAT MODULATE BOTH SEROTONIN AND DOPAMINE LEVELS)

As mentioned in Chapter 9, "Constant Craving," one of the biggest culprits in the Fat Wars is our difficulty overcoming unstoppable cravings. Many people cannot fight their physiological urge to binge eat, especially where insulin-spiking carbohydrates are concerned. It is important to recognize that in many cases the failure to lose excess fat may be largely due to various biochemical imbalances in brain chemicals that quite literally drive you to eat excessively. It is sometimes almost impossible to ignore the insatiable craving for these foods, and when we finally break down and give in we are greeted with a great big sigh that will most certainly only last an hour or two.

The pleasure (and fat gain) we often experience as a result of giving into these cravings is due to the rise in a brain chemical called serotonin (another chemical called dopamine can also rise in certain circumstances, further providing a reward feeling). As discussed in Chapter 9, serotonin is increased in response to insulin levels, and most of these "no-no" foods cause a drastic incline in this fat promoting hormone. When serotonin levels rise, we are greeted with instant gratification in the reward centers of the brain. Balanced serotonin levels are important in any fat-loss program because they provide a calming and appetite-suppressing action, which allows you to feel satisfied without needing to cheat.

Serotonin levels decline throughout the day and are replenished during the sleep phase. Many people who have sleep difficulties also have serotonin deficiencies. Serotonin levels are also quickly depleted during times of stress. And with the stressful lives we subject ourselves to day in and day out, it is not hard to imagine our serotonin tanks running on half empty at most times.

Listed below are nutrients that have been shown in studies to help control various (i.e., carbohydrate) cravings. I have listed only the ones that I feel may provide the greatest benefit to your fat-loss plan. These nutrients may be taken individually or combined for greater outcome (to simplify things, a complete formula called crave-free containing these as well as other co-factors is listed in Appendix I). These ingredients may also raise dopamine levels, which can also help control appetite.

WARNING: Those taking selective serotonin reuptake inhibitors, tricyclic anti-depressants, or monoamine oxidase (MAO) inhibitors should consult a health care professional before taking any of these ingredients.

- *Griffonia* – natural source of 5-hydroxytryptophan (5-HTP). Clinical trials have shown that supplementation with 5-HTP can safely reduce food cravings and promote weight loss. 5-HTP can boost brain serotonin levels due to its ease in crossing the blood–brain barrier and converting into serotonin.

- *Rhodiola rosea* – increases dopamine levels in the hypothalamus, an area of the brain governing appetite. This herb has also been well researched for its ability to help the body adapt to stress, which has been associated with food cravings in certain individuals.
- *Glutamine* – essential in brain function and especially important during times of stress. Glutamine has been used therapeutically to decrease cravings and addictive behavior.
- *Rhubarb root* – a number of published studies from China have demonstrated its use in weight-loss programs. Rhubarb supplementation has been found to be just as effective as the one-time anti-craving drug fenfluramine, but importantly without the side effects. Rhubarb leads to reduced food intake and increases a sense of fullness by decreasing stomach-emptying time.
- *Magnesium* – involved as a co-factor in over 300 enzymatic reactions in the body, including energy production through carbohydrate metabolism. Magnesium can help reduce cravings, particularly sugar and chocolate cravings in premenstrual women.

4. ANTIOXIDANTS

You may think it funny that I've added a section on antioxidants to a book on fat loss, but you'll soon learn why antioxidants help to play a role in burning your body fat. Without them, your chances of dropping the fat safely may be reduced.

Oxygen is a paradoxical substance. While oxygen is necessary for life, it can also harm cells. Antioxidants are produced by the body and are also present in many foods. They allow our cells to function properly by protecting us from free radicals, unstable molecules that can damage cell structures and lead to cell death. Free radicals are constantly being created by cell processes such as energy production, and by exposure to smoke, pollutants, solar radiation, and even aerobic exercise. Ninety-five percent of the free radical production takes place in our muscles' energy centers, the mitochondria (where fat is burned). So it is important to protect these energy centers from undue damage.

Free radicals are with us constantly. Scientists have identified 1,100 varieties of these cellular attackers to date. Recent research confirms that various antioxidants work together, each supporting the other in stopping cell-damaging free radicals in their tracks. Just as free radicals work in combinations, attacking us from every which way, antioxidants also work in synergy with one another to stop the onslaught.

Although there are perhaps hundreds of antioxidants, the ones that have been researched to be most effective as a family are vitamins C and E, alpha-lipoic acid (thioctic acid), reduced glutathione (GSH), and Coenzyme Q10 (CoQ10). These have been called the network antioxidants by Dr. Lester Packer and his group of researchers at the University of California at Berkeley. The network antioxidants work together as a team. The right combination of these antioxidants and other antioxidants not a part of the initial core team will contribute to your total cell health and maximum fat-burning ability.

Before you become overwhelmed by all the information on these various antioxidants and start to sweat just thinking of going out and purchasing them separately, don't worry. You can now easily find combinations of complete antioxidant formulas at your local health food store (the top one I recommend is protect, listed in Appendix I). I have listed an approximate daily quantity of each antioxidant in this section; however, this is only a guideline if you are deciding to take them separately (as opposed to a combined formula). The newest research supports taking your antioxidants together in synergistic combinations instead of separately.

Vitamin C

Vitamin C is a potent water-soluble vitamin. Its main job is to protect the watery interior of the cells. Vitamin C is also required for the production of the neurotransmitters, including serotonin. Over-fat and obese individuals, as well as those with Type 2 diabetes, require more vitamin C due to an increase in excretion rate. In addition, studies suggest vitamin C has a positive influence on cancer prevention, lowering the risk of cardiovascular disease, and improving collagen production. Because the body seems to reach a certain saturation point, it makes sense to take a smaller dose of vitamin C more often. Take 200 to 500 milligrams at a time, two to three times daily.

Vitamin E

Vitamin E is a terrific anti-aging antioxidant that improves the immune system, protects against sun damage, relieves arthritic symptoms, and makes strong cell walls. Vitamin E is a fat-soluble antioxidant, which means it can go places that water-soluble antioxidants, like vitamin C, can't. Two of the most important functions of vitamin E involve its action on fat-soluble structures, the cell wall itself, and the blood and cell-based fatty acids, which include LDL cholesterol and triglycerides (fats).

Under the age of 40: take 1–2 400 iu capsules a day of oil-based (mixed tocopherol) vitamin E, with food that contains some fat. Over the age of 40: take 1–2 400 iu capsules of dry-based (mixed tocopherol) vitamin E with food that contains some fat.

Lipoic Acid

Lipoic acid is amazing: It offers great protection against heart disease, stroke, memory loss, and cataracts. It also helps to control blood-sugar levels, reducing harmful blood protein-sugar complexes known as advanced glycation endproducts or AGEs. Its the AGEs that really put the age on diabetics because these persons are prone to making large amounts of this substance. So what's the problem with AGEs? They spin off gobs of free radicals that wreak havoc on cells, nerves, and connective tissue. This is a big reason why diabetics are at a super risk of kidney failure, blindness, and/or poor circulation. Lipoic acid is also critical for optimal energy production because it helps convert sugar (glucose) into usable energy for ATP re-synthesis, allowing your fat-burning cells to smile as they fire up the furnaces. It is recommended to start with 50 milligrams twice daily.

Take 50–100 milligrams of alpha-lipoic acid one to two times/day, approximately one-half hour away from food for best results. If you take over 100 milligrams, it would be wise to supplement with extra biotin (B vitamin), since high doses of lipoic acid may deplete this vitamin. If you are really exercising hard, smoke, or are exposed to a greater number of pollutants (i.e., the big city), you should up your consumption of lipoic acid to 100–150 milligrams twice daily.

Glutathione

Glutathione is the most important and abundant antioxidant naturally produced by the body. Through the bloodstream and the cells, it is perpetually neutralizing free radicals and removing toxins. Not only does glutathione boost the immune system, but research has shown that it also has an essential role in improved liver function, cancer prevention, promoting longevity, bronchitis, and psoriasis.

Pure glutathione in pill form has been shown to break down through digestion. The best natural way to boost glutathione levels in the body is to take lipoic acid and high-alpha whey protein isolates (see Appendix I for AlphaPure®). High-alpha whey proteins can contain up to 2.5 times the cysteine levels present in other whey protein isolates, which allows for an excellent and unsurpassed source of natural glutathione builders.

Coenzyme Q10

Along with vitamin E, Coenzyme Q10 (CoQ10) plays a free-radical defense role by riding along with lipoproteins in the bloodstream, protecting fatty acids from attack by free radicals (lipid peroxidation). Because energy is so very important in the proper functioning of your muscle cells, especially when it comes to disease prevention and burning fat, you'll want to take some supplemental CoQ10 to keep your mitochondria protected and your cells humming along nicely. Remember, a healthy active cell is a fat-burning cell.

CoQ10 is available as a powder or a gel form. CoQ10 can be expensive, but a small dose of 30–60 milligrams/day should do the trick without emptying your wallet. Take 30–60 milligrams/day of oil-based CoQ10 with foods that contain some fat.

Support Antioxidants

I've addressed the key antioxidants, but there are others that are also of great value to your antioxidant arsenal. These support antioxidants include selenium, zinc, manganese, and plant-based compounds called flavonoids. The flavonoids are of particular value as they can boost the effectiveness of vitamin C, glutathione, and the other antioxidants mentioned earlier. Berries such as bilberry, blueberry, and blackberry all contain valuable flavonoids, as does the spice turmeric, which has a potent antioxidant known as curcumin.

Note: I also recommend a good-quality full-spectrum B complex supplement each day, since the B vitamins are involved in the metabolism of proteins, carbohydrates, and fats, and a high-quality multi-mineral complex for added benefit (see Appendix I for recommendations).

Ephedra (Ma huang)

One of the most popular fat-loss supplements on the market is ephedra, also called Ma huang, a herb that contains the alkaloid ephedrine. Like *Citrus aurantium*, ephedra stimulates fat burning by activating beta-3 receptors. However, ephedra also activates other receptors, which causes the constriction of blood vessels and a rise in blood pressure. In January 2002, Health Canada requested a recall of products containing or recommending more than 8 mg per dose or 32 mg of ephedra/ephedrine per day, as well as of ephedra products recommending use for more than 7 days or ephedra products with stimulants such as caffeine.

If you have high blood pressure or are concerned about a rise in your pulse rate and blood pressure, you should be wary of Ma huang. Ephedra has pronounced medicinal qualities; coming from a plant in no way undermines its potency. If you decide to take ephedra, note that its effects are enhanced with exercise, and inform your doctor.

5. CITRUS AURANTIUM

Citrus aurantium is a natural stimulant that is derived from the essential oils of the bitter Seville orange. This herb has been used for thousands of years to improve circulation and liver function and to treat indigestion.

Increased resting metabolic rate means more fat calories burned. The fat-burning effect results from a group of compounds in the herb called adrenergic amines (organic compounds that are able to release or behave like adrenaline or noradrenaline), with the most effective one for fat loss being synephrine. Most extracts sold today are standardized for 4% or 6% synephrine. In addition to the flavonoids found in *Citrus aurantium*, this herb has the ability to produce an energizing and fat-burning effect on the body by activating a specific group of cell receptors known as beta-3 receptors. These receptors increase the rate at which fat is released from both fat and muscle cells (lipolysis), and increase the resting metabolic rate (thermogenesis). (You may even feel this herbal extract working, as your body will be generating heat.)

Citrus aurantium, unlike the popular fat-burning stimulant ephedra, does not raise pulse rate or blood pressure. The recommended dose of a standardized *Citrus aurantium* 6% synephrine extract is 325 milligrams/day, taken in divided doses about a half-hour before each meal or shake.

6. HYDROXYCITRIC ACID

A fruit from India called *Garcinia cambogia* contains an important fat-burning chemical called hydroxycitric acid, or HCA for short. While research has shown that HCA prevents the conversion of carbohydrates into fat, a more important function of this incredible nutrient is its ability to help increase the special fat-releasing enzyme called carnitine palmitoyl transferase (CPT). The enzyme that converts excess glucose into fat is called ATP-citrate lyase. HCA inhibits this enzyme from making more fat, and in the process slows down another enzyme called malonyl-CoA. The result is an increase in the levels of CPT (the fat-releasing enzyme).

HCA also inhibits glucose-stimulated insulin secretion, which helps to keep insulin in check. In the past, the HCA on the market was bound to a calcium salt, which may have inhibited absorption. Recently, a new HCA salt with magnesium (Mg) has come on the market. By adding Mg-HCA to your supplement program, you'll greatly increase your amount of CPT, which will allow for an increase in fat-burning potential. I suggest a dose of 500 milligrams to 2 grams of Mg-HCA derived from *Garcinia cambogia*, taken in divided doses twice daily, as a very important addition to your fat-burning army.

Chromium

As we've already discussed, high blood-sugar levels result in a spike in the hormone insulin, leading to cellular disruption and obesity. More than 90% of North Americans are deficient in chromium. Chromium is essential to reducing the cells' resistance to insulin. It helps your cells function better, allowing blood sugar and amino acids in and reducing blood-insulin levels. When you combine low chromium consumption with blood-sugar levels that are high due to a high consumption of sweets, breads, and refined foods, the result is a staggering increase in Type 2 diabetes, over-fatness, and obesity. Most soils contain little or no chromium. As a result, the plants we eat contain very little chromium. The best way to boost the level of chromium in your cells is to take a supplement.

Chromium is usually a very hard mineral to absorb effectively, but two of the most popular forms of chromium, chromium polynicotinate (niacin-bound chromium) and chromium picolinate, should both perform well and have been researched extensively. A recent study comparing the two forms of chromium in conjunction with exercise gave the nod to chromium polynicotinate. The recommended dosage is 200 to 400 micrograms of elemental chromium per day.

7. FORSKOLIN

Forskolin, from the herb *Coleus forskohlii*, increases the levels of the cellular messenger cyclic Adenosine Monophosphate (cAMP), which is a major regulator of fat-burning enzymes and a messenger that reacts with certain hormones to direct metabolic changes inside cells. Forskolin supplements are a must for anyone interested in boosting their fat-burning rate. Once cAMP is formed inside cells, it stimulates other enzymes that activate additional enzymes (a domino effect). As such, a little cAMP goes a long way; it is increased by high glucagon levels and reduced by high insulin levels. It also stimulates the thyroid hormones catecholamines and glucagon to perform their fat-burning jobs and other metabolic processes. Take a divided dose of 100 milligrams of *Coleus forskohlii* standardized to contain 10% forskolin (10 milligrams of forskolin) twice a day.

8. GREEN TEA EXTRACT

Green tea is beneficial for the mind and body, and can speed up fat loss. Tea is rich in flavonoids called catechins, which are very well absorbed by the body compared with other flavonoids. Catechins are powerful antioxidants and have been shown to inhibit certain cancers, improve blood flow in the cardiovascular system, and reduce LDL cholesterol oxidation.

Carnitine

Certain nutrients stimulate the actual fat-burning activity inside cells by activating the important enzymes required for the fat-burning process. Carnitine is one of them. Carnitine is part of the amino acid family, but works very much like a vitamin. It cannot, however, be classified as a vitamin since it is manufactured in the human body from two amino acids, lysine and methionine. L-carnitine is a natural substance essential for the mitochondrial oxidation of fatty acids; it regulates the energy metabolism of cells. Carnitine is a cofactor that helps transform long-chain fatty acids and then transports them into the mitochondria, where they are burned as fuel. Conditions that seem to benefit from supplemental L-carnitine include anorexia, chronic fatigue, cardiovascular disease, diabetes, male infertility, muscular myopathies, and obesity. L-carnitine also regulates the level of Coenzyme A (CoA) in mitochondria to ensure that energy metabolism is functioning at an optimal rate.

Carnitine is slowly absorbed from the intestines into the bloodstream, and the percentage absorbed is related to the amount ingested. The data tells us that the body can use just so much L-carnitine at one time. Ingesting carnitine at a dose of 1.5 grams twice daily can raise free carnitine by 20% and acetyl-L-carnitine by 80%. Carnitine is concentrated in human breast milk and colostrum (pre-milk breast fluid). Supplementing your diet with bovine colostrum may be a great way to increase carnitine levels.

Carnitine is also a part of the fatty acid transport enzyme carnitine palmitoyl transferase (CPT), which is needed to mobilize fat reserves for energy production. The trick to long-term permanent fat loss is to increase the amount and activity of CPT. Proper exercise can double CPT activity, making it a super-efficient catalyst in the fat-burning process. That is another great reason to train regularly. If you decide to add this nutrient to your Fat Wars team, you will need to take at least 500 milligrams of acetyl-L-carnitine or 1 gram of L-carnitine twice daily, on an empty stomach for best results.

In addition, recent research has shown the catechins in green tea to be thermogenic. Thus green tea extract may also help dieters shed fat, according to research in the December 1999 issue of *The American Journal of Clinical Nutrition.* This is the first human study to examine the influence of tea on energy expenditure and body composition. Green tea may be particularly useful for heart disease patients who are trying to lose weight because, unlike weight-loss drugs, it does not affect the heart rate. Catechin polyphenol compounds work with other chemicals to increase levels of fat oxidation and thermogenesis, helping the body burn fuels— such as fat.

If the fat-burning effect of green tea doesn't excite you, here are some other benefits: Green tea can lower serum glucose levels by inhibiting the activity of the starch-digesting enzyme amylase, so that starch is absorbed more slowly (insulin levels also decrease); it has also been shown to lower intestinal fat absorption. Diphenylamine, a compound in green tea, seems to have a strong sugar-lowering action as well. New research shows that green tea catechins produce one of the strongest vasodilating responses, thus allowing for increased blood flow. An increase in peripheral circulation is valuable for increased oxygenation and therefore increased energy production. If all this weren't enough, green tea also has the ability to raise brain levels of serotonin and/or dopamine, which control both the appetite and satiety response. Why not just drink green tea? Because standardized extracts of green tea have more of the active compounds than brewed tea alone can offer. I recommend taking 300–400 milligrams of green tea extract daily, standardized for 50% or more catechins, with a majority being one particular catechin called EGCG.

9. HGH SECRETOGOGUES

As mentioned in Chapter 2, the hormones of our body that regulate age and fat loss, HGH and the IGFs, decline by about 80% by retirement age. A secretogogue is a substance, chemical, or nutrient designed to encourage a gland to release a hormone.

As we go into middle age and beyond, the pituitary does not stop producing HGH; it just releases less of it into the bloodstream. A particular style of secretogogue can trigger the release of HGH, and in this way is able to bring about higher HGH levels than were occurring previously.

What this means is that, for a 40-year-old whose HGH levels have been on the decrease for about 20 years, a secretogogue can raise the concentration of HGH in the bloodstream to a more youthful level. In turn, this affords the possibility of halting or possibly even reversing some of the aging process and allowing the body to burn extra levels of body fat.

Because secretogogues cause the release of HGH from the body's own pituitary and at the body's own rate, the levels of HGH remain subject to governance by the hypothalamus and its feedback loop. Consequently, there is little or no possibility of artificially raising the serum levels of HGH to anything above normal, and consequently again, there is little or no possibility of bringing on serious side effects.

Another advantage to using secretogogues to achieve elevated HGH levels is that the cost of secretogogues is a fraction of that of injections. Also, with no needles involved, secretogogues can be taken at home without a medical presence on hand. Finally, because secretogogues are so safe, there is little monitoring required. In short, secretogogues are presently the safest, handiest, and most cost-effective means of elevating HGH levels in the body.

The initial research in this area was carried out by Dr. Daniel Rudman in a 1990 study published in the prestigious *New England Journal of Medicine*. The study tracked 26 men between the ages of 61 and 80 who were treated with HGH injections. Dr. Rudman, the lead researcher, presented astonishing results that showed that the majority of the participants experienced a 14.4% decrease in overall body fat, with an average 8.8% increase in lean muscle mass. The patients also experienced increased bone density, skin thickness, and skin elasticity. Dr. Rudman believed these changes to be equivalent to a 10- to 20-year decrease in normal aging.

A more extensive study was carried out at the Palm Springs Life Extension Institute, under the direction of Dr. Edmund Chein. This study, conducted between 1994 and 1996, involved 202 patients and employed hormone replacement therapy, chief amongst them being HGH. The results were striking. A study done in Rome in 1981 by Isidori and others showed that certain combinations of amino acid salts could stimulate pituitary HGH production dramatically when taken orally. Studies done with one secretogogue (SomaLife gHp) have shown a more than 800% increase in HGH production within half an hour of oral intake of 6 capsules.

Secretogogues are now used by most Longevity Medicine clinics throughout North America, either alone or in conjunction with HGH injections. They are a naturally effective way to elevate the fat-burning effect of your metabolism, and therefore increase your overall energy levels.

10. CONCENTRATED GREEN FOODS

Food is energy. This is a basic scientific principle. Your body is an energy system. Every single one of the 100 trillion cells in your body (little molecular motors) requires energy to work. Digestion, respiration, talking, seeing, hearing, circulation, thinking, metabolism—all require energy. When your body's energy is low, it just does not have the resources to run well, and that is when illness begins to dominate. When your energy is high, your peak performance and health are optimal. Food is the source of energy your body needs most. With precision and deliberate measure, nature has designed high-octane fuels for your energy support and biological functions.

Nutrition researchers have been telling us to eat our fruits and vegetables since we could remember. Fruits and vegetables contain phytonutrients (plant chemicals) that are capable of exerting powerful positive effects on our bodies. Even the simple soybean, or tomato, or blueberry, is a miracle of complexity far more intricate than the latest sophisticated computer program. It is recommended that we consume 6–10 servings of organic fruits and vegetables each and every day to obtain the maximum protection from these plant wonders. The reality, however, is that only a very small percentage of us actually do this. This is why concentrated green food powders are a smart addition to any health program, including *Fat Wars*.

Bio-energetic, whole plant–based foods are pure life energy. Grown in sunlight and infused with the energy of the soil and water, they can increase your energy, improve your moods, and help with continual fat loss. Look for only the highest-quality green food concentrates that contain both a mixture of organic land and sea vegetables and a mixture of synergistic herbs. High-quality powders can be mixed quite easily in a shaker cup (usually provided), and should be consumed either between meals or with a protein shake (a multi award-winning version of a green concentrate mixed with whey and soy protein isolates is listed in Appendix I).

KEY TACTICS

1. The right supplements make up for nutritional deficiencies in our foods.
2. Protein isolates are critical supplements in repairing and building healthy muscle cells.
3. EFA supplements ensure that you have the "right" kind of fat you need to burn the "wrong" kind of fat.
4. Crave-free supplements help to control unstoppable cravings, easing your ability to stay focused on the Fat Wars plan.
5. Non-stimulating metabolic enhancers (such as lean+) can increase fat-loss effects.

13

Getting Physical

Our bodies developed thousands of years ago. Back then, we walked, ran, and climbed to get where we were going and to secure what we needed. We fought for food alongside the many animals that shared our home. Today, it's a different story. We take our car to work, sit at a desk for hours, and then slump in front of the television each night. Boy, is life tough! It may well be mentally tough, but physically tough is another thing. We actually have to go out of our way to get physical.

Many people in this day and age suffer from obesity or over-fatness due to a very treatable syndrome called hypokinesis. Hypokinesis is just a fancy way of saying that a person lacks bodily movement. I've often said in my lectures that hypokinesis is as much at the core of obesity as is high insulin. Many studies have shown how ineffective a fat-loss program can be without proper exercise. In fact, exercise on its own, in many cases, can produce a sufficient loss of body fat (although fat loss is always more pronounced with a proper eating plan).

Our metabolism is designed to prepare for those times when we will be on the move. Our bodies save the fuel (fat) for a rainy day—a day that never seems to come anymore. In fact, fewer than 30% of North Americans engage in much physical activity, with the remainder of the population living life from one couch to the next. So we get fatter and fatter. Without proper fat-burning exercise, we will never win the Fat Wars.

While many of us value health and physical fitness, we have not learned to integrate physical activity into our daily lives. We all know people who exercise consistently, sometimes more than five times a week, week after week. They seem to be different from us. Instead of regarding exercise as a chore, they make it fun and invigorating, something that actually completes their life. For the rest of us, it's another matter. Most of us are great starters. We forge ahead at the beginning of the year, filling up the health clubs on January evenings to overflow capacity. But by April, it's business as usual. That health club membership is wasted, that piece of home exercise equipment gathers dust in the corner of the room, and that aerobics videotape is buried between *When Harry Met Sally* and *The Terminator*.

If we're going to lose as much fat as possible and keep it off, we have to get moving in the right way. However, the majority of exercise routines developed for weight loss over the past 20 years are not designed to melt away the fat and keep it off.

THE AEROBICS MYTH

Carmen had just turned 33, and with the births of three kids behind her, she felt ready to tackle her next task—dropping the fat that had slowly collected around her waist, hips, butt, and thighs over the past decade.

Exercise was nothing new to Carmen. She had already tried a variety of routines at the local community center. She had even ordered a few "miracle" devices from infomercials that seemed too good to be true. They were. Carmen tried walking, but the pounds just didn't seem to budge. She even invested in an abdominal-crunch machine and an aerobics video so that she could train at home. After three months of sweating to hip-hop, she felt more energetic, but the fat was still entrenched. What was she doing wrong, and why isn't she alone?

By far, the most common physical activity recommended for weight loss is aerobics. We've seen them: those spandex-clad cuties moving and shaking to the music, inviting us to get out on the dance floor and boogie with them. We've also seen the testimonials from those who have succeeded by adding aerobics to their weight-loss program. But the fact is that for every person who has won the war against fat by only using aerobics, there are 50 others who have not. The success rate when it comes to permanent fat loss via pure aerobics is not very high.

Many of us have tried aerobics ourselves. By aerobics, I mean any exercise that increases our body's need for oxygen. Most of us have gone running, spent what seemed to be hours on a treadmill or stationary bike, jerked our bodies to the music of an aerobics class or home video, and maybe even tried a Tae-Bo™ class or two. The truth is, many aerobic workouts are long, and the fat burned during the workout is minimal. As in dieting and fasting, the engines that actually burn the fat—muscle tissue—are burned up too, and the increase in the amount of fat burned before the next workout is almost zip. Hard-core aerobics is anti-muscle—athletes such as elite 10,000-meter runners or marathon participants carry very little muscle mass. Research confirms that excess aerobics causes overtraining and muscle wasting, with a subsequent reduction in fat burning.

Aerobics proponents have recognized this flaw, and many aerobic classes at gyms and health clubs these days also incorporate some sort of resistance training, such as taking steps (which uses body weight as resistance) or using small hand weights or elastic cords. But these attempts at making up for the deficiencies of most aerobic exercise are weak at best. Aerobic exercises—although they do have a role in your fitness regimen—are just not the most efficient fat-burning exercises.

BUILD MUSCLE, BURN FAT

In contrast to aerobics, resistance training builds muscle, and it's muscle that is going to help us win the war on fat. Not only do we want to build muscles, we want to turn on the muscles that we already have. Turn them on? Yes, the muscles we already have can actually be tuned up to become more efficient at burning fat. The right type of exercise can do that for us. We'll transform our muscles into the fat-burning army that they are capable of becoming. As the army ads used to say, "Be all that you can be." In this case, our muscles will burn all that they can burn.

Why are muscles so important? As I state throughout this book, muscles constitute the metabolic engine of the body. The more muscle you carry on your frame, the higher your basal metabolic rate (BMR), which refers to how many calories are produced during rest. And the more active those muscles are, the more fat you burn, 24 hours each day.

That fat we are packing around is deadweight. Fat is an inert substance—it just sits there taking up space (and it doesn't look that good either). Now here's the most important point—1 pound of active muscle can burn almost 50 calories a day. So, if you add muscle during your fat loss program, or at least keep the muscle you have, you will be well on your way to winning the Fat Wars. But too much cardio can quickly turn into a muscle-wasting activity. Common sense dictates, once again, that balance is the key. In this case, balance between resistance and cardio exercise.

In a landmark study published in the prestigious *American Journal of Cardiology*, aerobic training was compared with aerobic-with-resistance (weight) training. Participants were split into two groups and had to complete a 10-week exercise program. One group completed 75 minutes of aerobic exercise twice a week, while the other completed 40 minutes of aerobics, plus 35 minutes of weight training. At the end of the study, the aerobics group had an 11% increase in endurance, but no increase in their strength. The group that completed the combination of aerobics-with-resistance training showed a massive 109% increase in their endurance, and a 21% to 43% increase in their overall strength. Even though both groups spent the same amount of time exercising, the types of exercise they performed played a great role in their success. There are many other studies that further prove the theory that resistance training with low-impact cardio is superior to either one alone.

The usual scenario is as follows: You have been performing high-intensity cardio for weeks now, but you're no closer to reaching your fat-loss goals. In fact, you seem to have gained an extra pound in the last week. It's time to increase the cardio for better fat-burning effect. Bad move! The more cardio you do, the more likely your body will burn sugar and protein instead of fat. In order to create extra sugar, the body will begin to break down body proteins from muscle (remember gluconeogenesis from Chapter 10). Muscle will be lost, fat-burning capacity diminished, and the saga continues. This process cannibalizes muscle tissue almost faster than dieting does!

How Hard Do We Have to Work to Burn Fat?

In order to better understand how to train effectively for proper long-term fat-burning success, we first have to understand what type of fuel source the body uses to do specific activities. The problem is that most exercise primarily burns sugar and protein as fuel sources and leaves fat alone.

Sugars, as well as proteins, are broken down to their simplest forms for energy more easily than fat is. Fats are made up of many single units called fatty acids. These individual fatty acids must first be broken apart in order to contribute their energy value. Breaking down fatty acids is a lengthy process—and, as you saw in the discussion of metabolism in Chapter 1, many forms of exercise don't get us to fourth gear (the fat-burning one).

Most exercise programs touted by the exercise gurus of our generation tell people to train at 70% of their maximum heart rate for fat loss. The maximum heart rate is measured using that familiar mathematical equation of subtracting our age from the number 220. Training heart rate is calculated by multiplying maximum heart rate by the percentage we want to train at, in this case 70%.

> *Example:* Carmen is 33 years old, so she would calculate her training heart rate as: 220 – 33 x 70% = a training heart rate of 131.

The idea behind this training heart rate theory of 70% is that it will allow us to perform the most effective level of exercise—the one where our bodies are most apt to burn fat (referred to as the anaerobic threshold). But what the exercise gurus don't realize is that the closer we come to the anaerobic threshold, the further we move away from fat burning. In reality, this benchmark was never intended to measure fat burning. Instead, it was designed for cardiovascular fitness. Training at that heart rate will do wonders for increasing our heart and lung efficiency over time, but it won't do anything for emptying our fat reserves, at least not for the majority of people—those who have never trained at high intensity before.

If you haven't exercised in a long time or are unaccustomed to this intensity of exercise, the recommended training heart rate of 220 less your age times 70% will be much too strenuous for your fitness level. Your body won't be able to cope and you will start gasping for air. The minute this happens, the body switches gears and starts burning sugar as its main fuel. If you can't carry on a conversation while exercising without gasping for your next breath, then you're burning sugar instead of fat. Gasping is an indication that there is insufficient oxygen being supplied to the tissues. It takes an enormous amount of fuel to burn the dense fat molecules. When there isn't enough oxygen, your body is switching back to third gear (using sugar instead of fat). This is just one reason why people who engage in hour after hour, day after day of strenuous aerobics never ever seem to lose any fat. Imagine all that wasted time and effort!

Remember: Body fat is very dense and requires a great deal of oxygen in order to be burned as fuel.

You're thinking, "If fat needs a lot of oxygen, and we're all gasping for air in aerobics class, aren't we getting a lot of extra oxygen?" Yes and no! The problem is that we can never get enough oxygen when we are overexerting ourselves; that's why we're panting. As the intensity of the activity is increased, the availability of oxygen is actually decreased, because we're doing quick, shallow breathing to get air into our lungs, but we're not driving it deep enough. Our bodies have no choice but to switch gears and start mixing more and more sugar (and even amino acids from muscle) into the fuel mix.

The optimal intensity when it comes to fat loss is *whatever intensity allows us to take in enough oxygen to burn fat*. Usually it is much lower than the proposed anaerobic threshold of 70% and more like 50% to 60% of maximum heart rate. This is good news for all of you who love taking long walks, an excellent fat-burning exercise.

All this is laid out in more detail in Chapter 14, "The Fat Wars Action Plan"—don't worry if it seems confusing now.

How Long Do We Have to Work Out?
The length of time we perform an athletic activity can be just as important as the intensity the exercise is performed at.

Carmen arrives at the gym and starts her workout with aerobic activity. She punches in her usual 20-minute fat-burn routine on her favorite treadmill's computer, and away she goes. Exactly 20 minutes later, she hops off and allows the next confused, over-fat individual his turn. Within minutes, she's performing her usual weight-training routine, proud that she has already taken care of the fat-burning portion of her workout. After all, fat loss is her main objective; muscles can wait. But Carmen, like so many others, is mistaken not only about the ideal duration of the fat-burning portion of her exercise, but also about the order.

What is the optimum duration of cardio for effective fat loss? The answer may be surprising. We've all seen the signs posted in our local gym's cardio area: PLEASE RESPECT THE OTHER MEMBERS AND DON'T EXCEED 20 MINUTES ON THE MACHINES. But is 20 minutes enough time to burn fat? The answer, I'm sorry to say, is no!

Starting the Engine: If you live in a cold climate, then your first instinct after your butt hits the cold car seat is to turn on the heat. The problem is that there's no heat to be found; you just started the car, so it will take some time for the engine to warm up. Your body is like that freshly started engine when you begin to exercise—it needs time to warm up.

Fat fuel is not the starting fuel for cold bodies. The body usually starts warming up with a rich sugar mix instead. In order to change the primary fuel to fat, the body must first call into action hormonal and enzymatic responses. Remember: Hormones are those tiny, scurrying chemical messengers that give orders to the cells; enzymes are responsible for carrying out the orders. In this case, the adrenal glands start the ball rolling. Stress hormones (epinephrine) from these glands send messages out to the fat cells in order to get them to send some of their fatty acids into the blood. After these fatty acids are in the bloodstream, they are transported by special carrier proteins (discussed in Chapter 1) to the muscle cells. Specific enzymes further escort the fatty acids into the furnaces of those cells. This entire response (depending on a host of variables—undigested food, nutrients, etc.) usually takes at least 20 minutes to accomplish, which blows apart the theory of burning fat in the first 20 minutes. This means that just around the time we jump off the treadmill, our bodies have switched the fuel mix from sugar to fat. Too bad we're heading for the showers.

Keeping the Engine Revved: There are two things we can do to compensate for the 20-minute startup for effective fat loss:
- Do the cardio activity longer than 20 minutes to increase the fat-burning effect.
- Do the cardio activity after weight-bearing activity.

Well, the first is a no-brainer. We have already established that effective fat burning begins around the 20-minute mark of cardio exercise, so extending our workouts makes sense if fat burning is our goal. But what about the second? Why would performing cardio after weight-bearing exercise help fat loss?

A weight-training routine, performed correctly, is accompanied by a rush at the end of the workout. This high comes from a combination of endorphins (those pain-desensitizing chemicals that are even more powerful than morphine), anabolic hormones (testosterone and growth hormone), and stress-related chemicals (norepinephrine and epinephrine). Even though we are training primarily in an anaerobic fashion (without oxygen—the first three gears) and utilizing sugar as our main fuel source, we are still invoking a stress response that not only causes that incredible sensation after the exercise, but also frees up those fatty acids.

Doing cardio right after weight training is like getting into a car that has been running for a while. All we have to do is turn up the heat, and we get a blast of warm air. Our free fatty acids are now available to be burned through the cardio activity, right from the start. Now we can get off the treadmill after 20 minutes with the confidence that we have succeeded in burning body fat as our primary fuel source. This is especially true if our muscles have been used regularly and over a certain period of time. It takes, on average, about 15 days to convert your metabolism from a sugar-burning one to a fat-burner. Conditioned muscles utilize fat as a source of energy much faster than non-conditioned ones.

When Should We Work Out?

Now you know that intensity, duration, and sequence of exercises ultimately dictate what the fuel mixture will be during exercise; it takes 20 minutes to get to the fat-burning phase (a little less if we are conditioned). But when is the best time to perform exercise to maximize fat burning? The majority of us perform our exercise in the evenings. This is the time we walk into our local gym and have to take a number just to use the equipment. Exercising in the evening, usually after work, is wrong for two reasons.

- We are usually spent after a day of work and have little energy left for a workout. It's hard enough making dinner after work, let alone training. Our motivation at this time is usually low, and many people will come up with myriad excuses to avoid training. "I'm too tired, so I'll make up for it tomorrow by doing double." Sure you will, and while you're at it, why don't you complete my workout as well? The scary thing is that the increase in metabolic rate only lasts for the day the exercise is performed (unless you've succeeded in increasing your muscle size). So if we miss a couple of days of exercise, as far as metabolism is concerned, we are right back where we started: fat land.

* All of that incredible increase in our body's ability to burn fat for hours is shut down by sleep. And even though our sleeping metabolic rate (SMR) may be raised slightly, it hardly makes up for the rate at which we can burn fat while awake. Besides, in the evening our metabolism is at its lowest, readying our body for sleep. When we exercise late at night, we can offset this metabolic balance by secreting extra stress hormones, when they should be at their lowest. These stress hormones not only can keep us awake, but they also interfere with our recuperation process, ultimately slowing down fat loss.

The best time to exercise for the most effective fat burning is first thing in the morning. I know: You barely have enough energy to get out of bed in the morning, let alone hop on a treadmill. Over a short period of time (a few weeks), your body gets used to the new schedule, and before you know it, you can't believe you ever exercised at any other time of day.

Exercising in the morning allows you to take advantage of your body's higher metabolic rate for the entire day. Think about the possibilities. Every time you sit down to eat after exercising, your body is more efficient at burning the calories from the food you consume all day long. Unless you have no other choice, why would you want to lose this advantage by training at night? Besides, in the morning gyms aren't nearly as crowded. So what's stopping you from training at the most effective time for fat loss?

The Four Muscle-Building, Fat-Burning Exercise Rules

There are right and wrong ways to perform an exercise routine. If you follow the tips presented in this section, I guarantee that your progress will be greatly enhanced. These principles have been gathered from my extensive background in the fitness sciences field.

* Always warm up. A cold muscle is an inactivated muscle. It won't give you much performance, and it can be damaged if you push it too hard. Always take 10 to 15 minutes to warm up the body. Walking on a treadmill or peddling on a stationary bike are two good activities that will get the blood pumping. I do not recommend stretching right off the bat, since stretching a cold muscle can cause injury to that muscle. If you want to stretch, warm the muscle group first and then stretch.

- Technique is everything, especially when you're weight lifting. If I had a dollar for every time I saw someone training improperly, I'd be a millionaire by now. People seem to be in such a hurry when they work out, lifting weights improperly. Most of the time, these people don't even pay attention to the exercise they are performing. If you want to see results fast, then pay close attention to the way you perform your exercises. Do slow, controlled reps: Lift up smoothly and lower the weight to a count of two. The best advice I can give you is to remember that you are in control of the weight, not the other way around.

- Don't let your body become bored. Your body adapts to certain exercises rather quickly. If you keep doing the exact same exercises in the same order for any extended period of time (more than a month), your body will adapt and progress will come to an end. You have to keep your nervous system constantly guessing as to what exercises will be performed in what sequence. Research has proven that the body can begin to adapt to the same routine in as little as six sessions.

- Always cool down after completion. This is the opportune time to stretch. Take about 10 minutes at the end of the routine and cool down properly. When stretching, make sure you move into the stretch slowly, breathing deeply the entire time. Hold the stretch for at least 10 seconds (preferably 30 seconds to one minute) and then slowly come back to the starting position. Most people stretch improperly, which does nothing for the muscle except damage it. Stretching will also help to remove excess lactic acid that was produced during the weight-training phase of the workout.

Creatine, the Exercise Supplement

People having trouble adapting to resistance exercises or wanting to increase the effectiveness of their recovery time between workouts have tried a supplement called creatine.

Creatine is an important part of cell energetics. It combines with phosphates to make phosphocreatine (PC). PC replenishes lost, energy-rich phosphates that are used to make adenosine triphosphate (ATP), your cells' main energy currency. Creatine has been shown in many studies to increase muscle power in speed/strength athletes such as football players, sprinters, and weight lifters. Research also shows that creatine has a pronounced anabolic effect by increasing protein synthesis in trained muscles.

Creatine supplements can increase fat-loss results when accompanied by a proper weight-training routine. (This supplement is often used by body builders and power athletes who train with weights.) Creatine helps muscles work harder and recuperate faster by replenishing energy and stimulating muscle growth. Meat and fish are good natural sources of creatine—250 grams of meat contains about 1 gram of creatine. Taken as a supplement, 5 grams three times a day for men and two times a day for women for three or four days is sufficient to start. This is considered a loading phase designed to saturate the muscles with a lot of creatine. After the loading period, the daily dose is reduced to 2 to 5 grams a day, usually taken after exercise. It is best absorbed when it's mixed with a protein/carbohydrate shake after training (see Chapter 11). Creatine does not have to be loaded to be effective. A dose of 2 to 5 grams daily over several weeks works well and allows the muscles (and intracellular proteins) to recover from training and grow even faster.

The most common and affordable form of creatine is creatine monohydrate. Users may notice a slight weight gain from creatine monohydrate during the first two weeks of use. This is because creatine helps swell cells by increasing their water content. The extra water weight is a temporary phenomenon that is actually helpful in increasing the cells' anabolic activity.

Creatine works especially well when combined with the amino acids glutamine and taurine. Creatine can be purchased as a pure powder, or combined with other nutrients in a powder beverage. Either way, a 2- to 5-gram dose once daily after training could help exercising efforts.

Even though creatine has been shown to be generally safe, there are no studies on extended use. It is always better to err on the side of caution when taking cell-energetic supplements. Cycling the supplements is one way to be cautious. An example of a creatine cycle would be taking a daily dose (2 to 5 grams) for four to five weeks, and then taking a one-month break.

How Many Reps Should We Perform?

There is a distinct, scientifically proven set/repetition/intensity range that is most effective in muscular enhancement and muscle activity for long-term fat loss. Some experts believe that four to six reps per exercise builds the most muscle, others believe that 8 to 10 reps is the best way to go, and

still others believe you should strive for 15 and up. All this talk about repetition can be overwhelming to the novice exerciser, so in order to understand what a scientifically designed exercise routine should consist of, we
need to first take a look at the various muscle tissue in the body. You have
two kinds of muscle fibers: Type I (red) slow-twitch muscle fibers with a
high oxidative potential (red muscles are best suited for endurance), and
Type II (white) fast-twitch muscle fibers with a lower oxidative potential
(best suited for size).

- **Type I** slow-twitch muscle fibers use oxygen to produce a steady
  supply of energy. The fibers function more slowly than their fast-
  twitch counterparts and are best suited for non-intensive aerobic
  activities because they do not tire easily. These muscle fibers have
  large numbers of capillaries (small blood vessels) that are used to
  transport oxygen and nutrients into the muscle cells and remove
  waste products like carbon dioxide. Athletes who excel at endurance
  activities have a higher percentage of this type of muscle.

- **Type II** fast-twitch muscles do not have as high a need for
  oxygen, so they function well in an anaerobic (low oxygen)
  environment. These muscle fibers can contract rapidly, and do
  very well in high-intensity situations where strength and speed
  are needed. They are ideally suited for low-endurance activities
  that require quick bursts of energy, such as weight lifting,
  sprinting, or jumping. They are also called into use during
  many stop-and-go sports, such as basketball and volleyball. The
  fast-twitch muscle fibers tire quickly because of the increase in
  lactic acid, a by-product of anaerobic environments. Athletes
  who excel at short-duration, high-intensity activities seem to
  have a larger percentage of fast-twitch muscles.

These different types of fibers in the body require different rep sequences
to attain results. Slow-twitch fibers require many repetitions for maximum
effect, and fast-twitch fibers require a low to medium number of repetitions
for best results. Perform your exercises varying the rep sequences from 6 to 15.
The exercises could be performed in the following sequence: 1st set: 15 reps;
2nd set: 10 reps; 3rd set: 6 to 8 reps (this is just an example). Don't worry, I
have laid it all out for you in an easy-to-follow program in Chapter 14.

NEITHER TOO MUCH NOR TOO LITTLE

Too many people are much too concerned about the number of calories being burned during their exercise activities. By concentrating our efforts
on this aspect of training (see chart on page 172), it's easy to exercise too
long. That's right, we can do too much just as easily as we can do too little.

We need a little physical stress to increase the levels of free fatty acids, but too much can cause a drastic increase in cortisol, the muscle-wasting hormone. Dr. Barry Sears, best-selling author of *The Zone* series of books, warns against going over the 45-minute mark when it comes to weight training. Depending on our activity level, soon after 45 minutes the levels of cortisol (the major stress hormone) rise to the point where recovery from the exercise can become blunted. As you recall, cortisol is responsible for stealing valuable nitrogen from muscle tissue and turning the amino acids into sugar in order to create extra energy. The more cortisol that's produced, the harder it is to get rid of and the worse off we are for it.

We will never burn enough calories in the gym to make us happy anyway. What you may not realize is that the time you spend away from the gym can actually be more beneficial to your fat-burning efforts than the time you spend doing the actual exercise.

Cardio and weight-bearing activity won't burn a lot of fat during the exercise sessions themselves. The real magic lies in their ability to raise your resting metabolic rate (the rate at which you burn calories at rest). A great deal of this post-exercise activity is due to the rise in your anabolic hormones, testosterone and growth hormone, approximately 15 minutes after the exercise. As long as you don't blunt this metabolic increase by consuming the wrong foods afterwards, your body will have the ability to burn extra calories for many hours to come. As a matter of fact, in one study, it was shown that over two-thirds of the fat-burning activity of exercise takes place after the actual exercise sessions. This increase in fat-burning potential has been documented as lasting for over 15 hours in highly trained athletes.

When we complete our workout and are either on our way to work or plopped in front of the TV set watching our favorite programs, our bodies are still at work converting fat into energy. We know this because the post-exercise phase brings with it an increase in resting oxygen consumption and fat-burning enzyme activity. This means that after exercise you have an increased level of fat oxidation and an increased rate of triglyceride fatty acid cycling. Remember that fat is a very dense substance, requiring an enormous amount of oxygen and enzyme activity to annihilate it. Well, this increase in oxygen consumption and enzyme activity after exercise gives you the extra power you need to burn fat. In fact, in repeated blood-test studies in Sweden, the fat-burning enzyme (hormone-sensitive lipase) was elevated for a period of 12 hours after a one-hour walk.

Not only can you boost your fat burning after a workout, but you can also burn large amounts of fat while you sleep. The higher your sleeping metabolic rate (SMR), the more calories you burn during sleep. Exercise can increase your SMR by as much as 18.6%.

Calories Burned Having Fun

This chart gives you an idea of how many calories a 150-pound person would burn in one hour of the stated activity. You can see from the chart that you're probably not burning as many calories in the gym as you might hope.

When you do something you enjoy, you're often not thinking about the amount of calories being expended, but instead about the amount of fun you're having. Ultimately, doing something that you think is fun is the best way to burn calories on a regular basis.

Activity	Calories Burned Per hour
Aerobic exercise, moderate intensity	350
Bicycling or stationary cycling (10 mph)	415
Hiking with a 20-pound backpack (3 mph)	400
Roller skating	350
Dancing	350
Treadmill walking (4 mph)	345
Calisthenics	300
Rowing machine, low intensity	300
Rowing machine, moderate intensity	655
Golf, walking with clubs	270
Walking, mild (2 to 2.5 mph)	185 to 255
Walking, vigorous (5 mph)	555
Stair-climbing machine	680
Rope-jumping	660
Step aerobics, moderate intensity	610
Cross-country skiing (5 mph)	600
Swimming	540

SHOULD I EAT BEFORE EXERCISING?

Any way you look at it, exercising is stressful on the body, which is why the body responds by elevating certain stress hormones (i.e., adrenaline and cortisol). When the body is stressed, it doesn't prioritize digesting food. Most of the blood supply is escorted to the extremities, not the stomach. This is why you should not consume a lot of solid food before exercise; it will just sit there fermenting in your gut. You should train yourself to exercise on an empty stomach, or only consume between 100 and 150 calories about 30 to 45 minutes before exercising. If you do eat something prior to working out, carbohydrates aren't the best choice, due to their insulin-raising ability, which causes you to use glucose (sugar) as your primary fuel instead of fat.

If you consume protein in the form of an easily digestible whey isolate, the protein will empty from the stomach quickly. It will also cause a rise in the hormone glucagon (the primary hormone for maintaining glucose levels during exercise), allowing for enhanced fat-burning activity. So if you must eat something before exercise, make it a protein shake with water, and keep it to around 100 calories (my favorite pre-exercise shake is one full serving of transform+ with water).

What About After?

After any athletic activity, especially weight training, the body requires refueling of its glycogen (short-term energy) reserves. In order to ensure that this happens, the body contains an enzyme called glycogen synthetase that is responsible for storing sugar for future needs. Within a two-hour window after exercise, this enzyme is extra hungry. This two-hour window is the only time that you can consume larger-than-normal amounts of carbohydrates without worrying that they'll convert to fat.

Many of us make the mistake of consuming only carbohydrates after a workout (fruit juice, etc.). Drinking carbohydrate beverages without consuming sufficient protein after exercise causes a drastic increase in insulin levels. The insulin spike depresses growth hormone and testosterone levels. New research presented in *The Journal of Physiology* in 2001 confirms that protein mixed with carbohydrates soon after training allows for faster muscle recovery and greater growth hormone and testosterone increases.

As close to the completion of your workout as possible, mix protein with carbohydrates in a liquid form to ensure rapid replacement of bodily sugars and protein for recovery. The post-workout protein should be primarily in the form of an isolated whey protein that's high in alpha-lactalbumin for maximum timing and absorption value. The carbohydrates should come from mixed whole fruits, primarily from the berry family due to berries' superior antioxidant-carrying capacity.

BECOMING A GYM RAT OR STAYING HOME GROWN

A health club or gym is a really great place to get physical, but it's not for everyone. The advantages of a gym include the large variety of equipment to choose from; the atmosphere, which can be social and uplifting; and the fact that there's often expert help in the way of a certified trainer to help keep you on the right path. A gym allows the use of a variety of free weights and weight machines that usually aren't available at home. In a gym, you can set up a weight circuit, using free weights or plate-loaded machines, which allows you to move from one exercise to another very efficiently. Also, you can hire a personal trainer for one or more sessions to help you perfect your weight-lifting technique. (A personal trainer will cost you some more money, but it may be well worth the price, especially if you're a novice at weights.)

The downside is that a gym costs money. A gym membership will run anywhere from $35 to $100 a month, and sometimes more for the fancier clubs. In addition, some people feel self-conscious going to a gym—at first glance, everyone else looks buffed, toned, and tanned. It's a little intimidating when Biff, the gym rat, moves into your space and gives you a stare as if to say, "What are you doing in my gym?" Also, working out at a gym can take a little more time than working out at home. There's travel to get there, the workout, shower, and travel home. That can add an extra hour to an already busy day, which might present another excuse for not exercising.

Don't get me wrong. I think the advantages of a gym far outweigh the disadvantages, but the most important thing is to get on the right path to winning the Fat Wars by increasing your level of physical activity any way you can.

A word of caution is in order. If you do join a gym, do not let a trainer talk you into doing a traditional bodybuilding routine, or, because you are over-fat, recommend that you hit the treadmill for an aerobic blast. The trainer's role should be just to show you the various weight-bearing exercises and how to perform them properly and safely.

Fitness on the Go

If you travel, plan on keeping up with your exercise program while on the road. If you can't get a hotel with a gym, you can still figure out a way to do a variety of exercises, some of which may be with resistance, in an interval fashion.

Special vinyl dumbbells are available that can be filled with water. You can pack them in your suitcase and take them along on your trip, and then fill them up for a quick workout in your hotel room. Elastic bands also can work well (these are what I use when I can't find a gym). Remember: Everything counts! A little workout is better than nothing, especially if you are eating out a lot and need to burn the extra calories that restaurant food typically contains. (You could always leave some of it on the plate.)

While there are dozens of exercises you could do, I prefer the basic lifts—they are easy to do and stimulate the greatest amount of muscle in the least amount of time. As gym memberships go, try to work out a deal with the club. Buy a three-month membership to see if gym training is right for you. Even if you decide to train at home later on, you won't be out a lot of cash.

If you do feel intimidated and self-conscious training at a health club, just remember that others training alongside you will respect you for doing it. They know that what you're trying to accomplish is something that millions of couch potatoes are avoiding. No one will make fun of you or condemn you for fighting the good fight. Look around very carefully; there are just as many—if not more—people there who look just like you as there are people who look like professional athletes. (Where I work out, hard bodies are on the endangered list. The toned, tanned, and buffed stand out like sore thumbs because there are so few of them.)

If you can't afford a gym membership, or you're too intimidated to train with others, or it takes too much of your time, or you just like to train by yourself, then consider training at home or in the great outdoors. You don't have to use the fancy equipment found in a gym for great results, although I think it helps. You can buy an inexpensive barbell set or a set of adjustable dumbbells from your local mass retailer or sporting-goods store for under $60. You can also use other items around your house, such as a couple of old cans (from soup to paint, as you become fitter).

BE ACTIVE ALL DAY LONG

Every little bit helps. The more active you are throughout the day, the more fat you will burn. Activity increases the body's ability to utilize calories. Every time you take the stairs instead of the elevator, every time you choose a parking space a little farther from the mall, and every time you play with your kids instead of saying "I'm too tired" counts!

We should not limit activity to formal exercise. While we want fat-burning exercise to be our main means of transformation, other kinds of physical activity will also keep our metabolism high. After all, every little bit helps when we're making progress in the Fat Wars.

GOING FORWARD

If you truly want to lose fat and keep it off for life, you know what has to be done. Exercising regularly is definitely the smart thing to do if you want permanent weight loss, but there are some specific ground rules that can lead to success or failure. Here they are:

- Don't expect to transform your body overnight. We seem to forget the road that got us here in the first place. We didn't wake up one morning to suddenly discover layers of fat on our formerly buff physiques. We got here one Twinkie at a time. It all adds up. Give yourself sufficient time to reach your goals, an ounce of fat at a time.

- What you did in the past doesn't count. You may be skeptical about whether this new information on exercise will work for you. You may have tried physical activity before, only to see no results and drop out. The improvements just weren't worth the effort. That's all about to change. If applied correctly, you will lose fat, and lots of it. This is true for everyone—men, women, and children—regardless of how over-fat you are.
- Get into the Do Zone. The words on these pages will not burn your fat. You will burn your fat. You must become self-motivated to succeed. The best way to get into the habit of regular exercise is through plenty of practice, beginning with the exercises outlined in the Fat Wars 45-Day Transformation Plan in Chapter 14.
- Take an honest look at the reasons why you stop yourself from exercising. Don't beat yourself up for not getting physically active, but don't put all the blame on your situation. There will be times that are out of your control when you won't be able to exercise. But more often than not, something that prohibits you from training is just in your mind. Don't put off exercise for one more minute.

Apply the strategies you've learned here as if they were the last detail of your fat-loss battle plan, because they are. Without exercise, you will fall short of your objectives. And even if you lose weight, you will likely gain it all back, and then some. Is that what you really want? Or would you rather lose the fat and keep it off permanently? I thought so.

KEY TACTICS

1. Aerobic exercise on its own is not an effective long-term fat burner.
2. Resistance training builds muscle, which is critical to burning fat.
3. Do not lift weights for more than 45 minutes at a time.
4. Morning workouts are best for fat burning, as they increase metabolism for hours afterwards.
5. Be active and work out regularly, wherever and whenever you can.

14

The Fat Wars
Action Plan

This chapter is designed to help you develop your personal Fat Wars 45-Day Transformation Plan. Why 45 days to transformation? As I mention in Chapter 13, it takes at least 15 days to convert your body from a sugar-burning machine to a fat-burning one. In my experience, it generally takes at least another 30 days before you can notice a significant change in how you look, feel, and perform. Remember: This is not a get-lean-quick scheme! Dedication and hard work are required to change a lifestyle that has probably been with you for a very long time. Nothing happens overnight; something as important as life transformation occurs through numerous small steps.

In this plan, 45 days to transformation really means nine weeks. The plan is broken up into nine five-day cycles, starting on Monday and ending on Friday. This doesn't mean that on the weekends you can forget all the changes you've made. Instead, the five-day cycles are designed to give your body a chance to adapt to the stimulus of the resistance and cardio exercises and your new way of eating. You can choose to continue your aerobic exercise on the weekends by walking or doing some other low-impact activity, or you can choose to take a break from any exercise; it's really up to you. Your body knows what's best—sometime it will want a rest to recover from a tough week; sometimes it will want to get out there and play. Listen to your body, and whatever you choose, staying close to your new eating strategy throughout the nine weeks (yes, this means weekends too) is very important.

Make a genuine commitment to sticking with the program for nine weeks. Forty-five days isn't that long a period to establish new habits for a healthier, fitter future. I have received hundreds of testimonials from people who were at first reluctant to begin the transformation period of the Fat Wars plan. The letters say how glad the people are that they stuck to it, and how quickly the time passed. These people have completely turned their lives around. Forty-five days is nothing when it comes to a life change. The way you will feel at the end of the first 45 days will amaze you, not to mention those around you. In the long run, you will change your life as well as your body.

Think of this image. A stone is placed in one pan of a scale. The stone keeps the pan down, but a fine trickle of sand in the other pan will eventually start to lift the stone, then it will balance the stone, and eventually outweigh the stone—even if it seems that the sand is having no impact at first. In our lives, the sand is every effort we make at self-improvement, no matter how small. As long as the sand keeps pouring (as long as we keep working) the stone will eventually be lifted.

Your excess body fat can be viewed as your stone, and the little changes you make every day during the 45-day transformation period can be seen as the sand. Before you know it, the stone has been lifted and you are a new, improved version of your former self. But once the excess fat has been lifted, you must maintain your new lifestyle so that the fat never returns. You must remain committed to your new lifestyle and never look back. Luckily, good health is addictive.

THE BEST TIME TO CHANGE

Fat Wars was written to give you a scientific approach to changing the way you look, feel, and perform. It is in your best interest not to put this change off any longer—start changing your habits today. Change is one of the hardest things to accomplish; it's hard to break out of old habits. We all get caught up in our own little comfort zones because they are familiar, even though we know that we need to create new habits and new patterns.

Failure, believe it or not, can also be something we are comfortable with. If you've been overweight most of your life, even though you may want to change on some level (probably a very deep one), being overweight may be a part of your comfort zone. If you were to shed your fat, you would be on unfamiliar ground; you would look, feel, and perform differently— better—than you've ever dreamed. Instead of seeing this as a scary prospect, accept that the change will be an exciting one.

THE FAT WARS 45-DAY TRANSFORMATION PLAN

During the first 45 days of the rest of your life, some positive changes will set the stage for permanent fat loss. Cell sensitivity to insulin will increase, reducing resting levels of insulin, blood fats, and glucose. This increased sensitivity will make your muscle cells happy and ready to work for you by burning fat.

During the 45-day period, your body will try to adapt to the extra stimuli from the resistance and aerobic portions of the exercise component, and muscle growth and vital capacity (your body's ability to utilize oxygen) will increase. In men, this will mean an increase in muscle mass and strength, as well as an increase in transport proteins, fat-burning enzymes, and immune factors. Women will experience these benefits, but without the bulk gains that men experience. Levels of cortisol (the muscle-wasting hormone) will begin to drop and levels of glucagon (the fat-releasing hormone) will rise. While you will burn fat, remember that you will be building muscle, which weighs more. Look for a leaner, but not necessarily lighter, figure in the mirror.

Don't become discouraged in the first few weeks—you are bound to lose some battles in the Fat Wars. Your body has become accustomed to the extra fat that covers the leaner you underneath, so at first it may be reluctant to change. Just keep on plugging away, and in 45 days you will be amazed at your progress. Remember that at least two weeks will probably pass before you notice a change in body shape (for some, this can seem like the longest two weeks of their lives), but changes in mood may happen within the first week.

Make a full commitment to yourself to complete the Fat Wars 45-Day Transformation Plan and to stick to the recommendations as closely as possible. Take stock of what you're eating now. Make a commitment to assess your diet, and start to buy and eat more healthy food, consuming five meals a day (three solid meals and two shakes). Take a step-by-step approach to making these new and healthful habits part of your life.

In Chapter 13, you learned what type of exercises to perform and how to do them for maximum effect. Now's the time to put this into action. If you have never trained with weights before, it would be a good idea to hire a personal trainer to take you through the first week of the Fat Wars 45-Day Transformation Plan (see *www.fatwars.com* for a Fat Wars trainer in your area). Please stick closely to these exercises and their format. The routine was designed to make sure that you see results within the 45 days.

The supplements that I recommend in this book can be added at any time during the plan, but including them right from the start is best. This plan was not designed to burn you out, so don't burn the candle at both ends. Get plenty of rest and allow yourself enough time for the deep sleep that restores your body so that you can continue to progress. Don't forget that rest gives your body a chance to rebuild itself (deep, delta, slow-wave sleep releases the most HGH). Remember that after the first 45 days, you won't want to look back! Follow this step-by-step strategy, and say hello to the new you!

CRAFTING YOUR FAT WARS FOOD PLAN

The Importance of Water

When it comes to increasing our overall health, we often forget to increase our consumption of one of the most important elements of all—water. Water is essential to the biochemical functions of the human body (we are, in fact, mostly water!). Your bones are one-quarter water. Your brain and muscles are three-quarters water. Your blood and lungs are over 80% water. Next to oxygen, water is the most important ingredient of life. Then why don't the majority of us drink enough of it? Well, you might say, "I drink plenty of liquid: juice, coffee, tea, sodas." But nothing can take the place of water. Indeed, many of us may be dehydrated and not even know it!

Increasing your water intake while you exercise is imperative, because water is vital in cardiovascular function and temperature regulation. As you exercise, your muscles create a lot of extra heat. The heat is transported through tiny blood vessels, called capillaries, that are near the surface of your skin. The release of perspiration from your sweat glands and sweat's evaporation has a cooling effect on the skin and on the blood in the capillaries beneath it.

Sweating is an essential mechanism in your body's cooling system. If your body doesn't have enough water to make this system run smoothly, your blood-carrying capacity diminishes. Don't forget: Blood's role is to carry nutrients such as oxygen, glucose, fatty acids, and proteins to the muscles to create energy. The blood must also remove the toxic residue of metabolism, such as carbon dioxide and lactic acid. Since your circulatory system is almost 80% water, the extra demand for water can be quite severe. Intensive exercise can cause a person to lose 5 to 8 pounds of fluid through perspiration, evaporation, and exhalation. Studies show that as fluid is lost, the efficiency with which the body produces energy drops significantly. Try to consume clean, filtered water throughout the day.

Losing excess fat can also cause a release of toxins into your body, since many toxins are lodged in the fatty tissue. Water is essential in the detoxification process, and since you will be dropping fat, you will need all the water you can drink.

In his best-selling book, *Your Body's Many Cries for Water,* Dr. Fereydoon Batmanghelidj suggests that somewhere during our evolution, the signals for thirst and hunger may have become the same. Dr. Batmanghelidj believes that often when we think we are hungry, we are, in fact, just thirsty. In order to cut down on the impulse to overeat, I recommend that you drink a glass of water about 15 minutes before eating. This way, you will be guaranteed not to overeat to satisfy an urge for water intake.

Carry your water with you everywhere you go (I even bring my water to bed) in a closed container, and drink it through a straw to avoid swallowing excess air. One of the biggest reasons people do not consume enough water through the day is that they drink the water from a glass and end up gulping excess air that bloats their stomachs. Drinking from a straw avoids this problem.

How Much Can You Eat in a Day?

For best results on the Fat Wars 45-Day Transformation Plan, you will have to figure out your total daily calorie allotment. Remember that if you take in more calories than you burn throughout the day, the excess will end up as winter insulation. Following are two methods that you can use to figure out your daily caloric needs. Method 1 was developed for those individuals who aren't crazy about following strict guidelines. Although the simplicity of Method 1 is appealing, Method 1 is not as effective as Method 2, which gives explicit directions on how to calculate your daily calories and individual macronutrient portions. The best method to use is the one you will stick with throughout the 45-day transformation period. So pick one and stay as focused and as committed as you can for the duration of the program.

If you would like to download a detailed list of foods and their individual values of calories per portion and grams of protein, carbohydrates, and fat per portion, please visit the Fat Wars Web site at *www.fatwars.com* and click on the Fat Wars Fuel icon.

Method 1: The Simple Simon Method

Many people who have come to my seminars or who have read *Fat Wars* have told me that they were unable or didn't want to follow the nutrient-counting part of the plan, but still experienced significant fat loss. This is because many of the recommendations in *Fat Wars* are common-sense suggestions on how to lose fat. If you exercise regularly, eat smaller portions of food five times a day, and make sure these meals are metabolically balanced, you will lose body fat—only not as fast or effectively as you will if you stick to the dietary advice in this section.

If you're not one who believes in weighing your food and calculating your daily caloric allotment, that's okay. You can still make the Fat Wars plan productive by following these guidelines:

- Re-read Chapters 6 through 8 to find out what your best food choices are on the Fat Wars plan.
- Never let more than three-and-a-half hours pass between meals.

In addition, eat five meals every day: three solid meals and two protein shakes. Each meal should contain protein (30%), essential fats (30%), and low-glycemic carbs (40%). Of course, in this instance you would use approximate values. The last meal should be void of any high- or medium-glycemic carbs, with best results coming from various forms of lettuce.

Attention night-shift workers: If you work the night shift, the last meal you consume prior to sleeping should be void of any high- or medium-glycemic carbs.

Here are some tips to help you create a Fat Wars meal:
- Use a dinner-sized plate and visually divide it into three equal sections.
- Use the palm of your hand to determine the size for your protein element. Place the protein in one of the sections on the plate. For example, you could eat a serving of chicken or turkey that's roughly the size of your palm.
- Fill the other two-thirds of the plate with a heaping portion of fresh fibrous vegetables for the carbohydrate portion. If your carbohydrate choice is a starch (and starches should be limited during the 45 days) such as a sweet potato, rice, or beans, add only one-third more than the protein portion, for a 1.3 to 1 ratio (see "No Wheat, No Rice," page 187).
- For your fat source, use about half your palm as a measurement. If you choose seeds or nuts, use the half-palm measurement; or use one tablespoon of olive or flax oil and drizzle it over vegetables or salad. If your protein choice contains fat, such as red meat or fish, drizzle only a small portion (no more than a teaspoon) of organic olive oil over the meal or simply add a few almonds.

Note: The above method is very basic. Calculating your individual caloric allotment and macronutrient portions during the 45 days is always a better method and produces greater results, even though it may seem tedious at first. After the 45 days, you will definitely have a better grasp of how many calories and what type of calories to consume to keep you on the winning side of the Fat Wars if you follow Method 2.

Method 2: The Serious Approach
Over the last year, I have received hundreds of letters and e-mails from people who followed the Fat Wars 45-Day Transformation Plan. I've heard all sorts of success stories—especially from people who followed Method 2. With this method you leave very little to chance, which allows for greater success on the program. Method 2 is a strategic plan of attack on your 30 billion fat cells, and based on hundreds of testimonials, it is your best chance for success.

As you have probably figured out by now, protein is the Four Star General that leads the army in the Fat Wars. After first figuring out your daily protein needs (in calories or grams), you can then calculate the remaining calories or grams of the other two nutrients (fats and carbs). In order to receive a reliable assessment of your daily protein needs, you will first have to get a lean body analysis completed. If you do not have access to one of the body fat analyzers that I recommend on my Web site *www.fat-wars.com*, then use the tables below to find your body-fat percentage. Although not as accurate as a professional method, the tables are a close enough guideline to follow.

Directions: Find your height on the left of the chart, then look for your present weight: The intersection is your rough body-fat percentage.

Average Male

Height	Weight										
	150	160	170	180	190	200	210	220	230	240	250
5'6"	17	19	21	23	25	27	29	31	33	35	37
5'7"	16	18	20	22	24	26	28	30	31	33	35
5'8"	14	15	18	20	22	24	26	28	30	32	33
5'9"	12	14	16	18	20	22	24	26	28	30	32
5'10"	10	13	13	16	18	20	22	24	26	28	30
5'11"	9	11	13	15	17	19	20	22	24	26	28
6'	8	9	11	13	15	17	18	20	22	24	26
6'1"	8	9	10	12	14	16	18	19	21	22	24
6'2"	8	7	9	11	13	15	17	19	21	22	23
6'3"	8	7	8	10	12	14	16	18	20	21	22
6'4"	8	7	7	9	11	13	15	17	19	20	21

Average Female

Height	Weight										
	100	110	120	130	140	150	160	170	180	190	200
5'	23	26	29	36	40	44	46	48	50	50	50
5'1"	21	24	26	34	38	40	44	46	49	50	50
5'2"	18	20	26	32	35	39	42	46	49	50	50
5'3"	17	22	25	32	33	36	40	43	46	49	50
5'4"	16	26	28	30	31	32	34	36	38	42	46
5'5"	16	20	26	28	30	32	34	36	37	40	43

Height	Weight										
	100	110	120	130	140	150	160	170	180	190	200
5'6"	16	22	24	26	28	30	32	34	35	40	42
5'7"	16	15	20	22	24	26	28	30	32	34	37
5'8"	16	15	18	20	22	24	26	28	30	32	34
5'9"	16	15	18	18	20	22	24	26	28	30	32
5'10"	16	15	18	18	18	20	22	24	26	28	30

Once you have determined your body-fat percentage, take the number and subtract it from your present weight. The new number represents your lean body mass. Now you can calculate your daily protein requirements. Use the formula that best describes your activity level:

- **No Exercise:** 0.75 x lean body weight (in pounds)
- **One to Two Workouts Per Week:** 1.00 x lean body weight (in pounds)
- **Over Three Workouts Per Week:** 1.15 x lean body weight (in pounds)
- **If You Are an Athlete:** 1.25 x lean body weight (in pounds)

The number that you get represents your daily protein requirement, in grams, on the Fat Wars plan. Take this number and divide it by five to arrive at the amount of protein allotted at each meal.

I'll use one of my clients, Lisa, as an example:

- Step One: Lisa presently weighs 150 pounds and carries 30% body fat. If I multiply 30% (which is equal to 0.3) by 150, I end up with the number 45, which represents the total amount of fat in pounds she is carrying (.30 x 150 = 45 pounds).
- Step Two: Because fat is an inert substance, it doesn't require any protein, unlike our lean body mass. So next, I subtract the amount of body fat (45 pounds) from Lisa's present body weight (150 pounds) and I arrive at 105 pounds of lean weight.
- Step Three: I then take 105 (Lisa's lean weight) and multiply it by 1.15 since Lisa has just started the Fat Wars plan (105 x 1.15 = 121).
- Step Four: The number 121 represents Lisa's total daily protein requirement in grams.
- Step Five: Because she is following the Fat Wars plan and is now eating five times per day, Lisa now divides 121 grams by 5 meals to get 24 grams of protein per meal.
- Step Six: Lisa would now make sure that each of her five meals throughout the day contains approximately 24 grams of protein.

After you have your total daily requirement of protein, you can easily figure out your total caloric allotment by following these guidelines.

- **Total Protein Calories (30%):** Take your total daily protein requirement, in grams, and multiply this number by 4 (which is the calorie per gram value of protein). Using our example, Lisa would multiply 121 by 4 (121 x 4 = 484 calories of protein per day).
- **Total Fat Calories (30%):** Your total fat calories must come as close as possible to your total protein calories. Lisa's ideal intake of fat calories would be 484 calories per day. In order to arrive at the total amount of fat in grams that you should eat per day and per meal, you then divide 484 (or whatever your number is) by 9, which is fat's calorie per gram number. Lisa's equation would look like this: 484 ÷ 9 = 54 grams of fat per day. To find the amount of fat in grams per meal, simply divide the total number of fat grams by 5, which is the number of meals you want to eat each day. Keeping to our example: 54 ÷ 5 = 11 grams of fat per meal.
- **Total Carbohydrate Calories (40%):** Since carbohydrates should be about 40% of your total calories, you simply multiply your protein requirement in grams by 1.3. Lisa's equation looks like this: 121 x 1.3 = 157. The total number of carbohydrates, in grams, that Lisa is allotted per day is 157, or 31 grams per meal (157 ÷ 5 = 31). For Lisa to figure out the caloric value, she would take 157 and multiply it by 4, as each gram of carbs has 4 calories: 157 x 4 = 628. Lisa is allotted 628 total carbohydrate calories per day, or almost 126 carbohydrate calories per meal (628 ÷ 5 = 125.6).
- Now add up the total caloric values from your three macronutrients (protein, fat, and carbohydrates) to arrive at your total caloric intake for each day on the Fat Wars program. Lisa's total daily caloric value would be almost 1,600 calories per day (484 protein cal. + 484 fat cal. + 628 carbohydrate cal. = 1,596).

For the best results, you should try to hit that caloric value as closely as possible each day.

Note: Please understand that Fat Wars is not a starvation diet plan in any way. The plan is based on lean body percentage and active tissue (lean body mass) caloric needs. There's no point taking in more calories than you are going to burn if your goal is fat loss. If you are a larger and more active participant than my example of Lisa, you will have a larger calorie allotment. The reverse is also true.

This is a plan that you should adhere to for nine straight weeks; after that, your needs will change, just as your body does. The reason this plan is so effective is that it does not promote hunger, due to the balancing of the three macronutrients. If you wish to increase your caloric values on the weekends, that's up to you, but stick within the 40-30-30 Fat Wars macronutrient profile. The best results are found by sticking as close to your caloric values as possible for every day of the nine weeks.

Finding Your Macronutrient Meal Profile Another Way

Total calories per day, based on your present lean body body weight and activity	Multiply by	Divide by the number of calories per gram	Divide by the number of meals per day	Macronutrient profile (in grams)
	.40	4	5	Carbohydrates per meal
	.30	9	5	Dietary fat per meal
	.30	4	5	Dietary protein per meal

For example, Lisa at her present 150 pounds has used the quick method to calculate that her daily calorie intake should be 1,600 to achieve her fat-loss goals. Her chart will look like this:

Total calories per day, based on your present lean body body weight and activity	Multiply by	Divide by the number of calories per gram	Divide by the number of meals per day	Macronutrient profile (in grams)
1,600	.40	4	5	32 grams carbohydrates per meal
1,600	.30	9	5	11 grams dietary fat per meal
1,600	.30	4	5	24 grams dietary protein per meal

Your main objective here is not to go over your allotted number of calories each day for the 45 days. It doesn't matter if you are off slightly from day to day in your grams per meal or total figures. Remember that protein is the macronutrient responsible for up-regulating your metabolism, so try to be stringent in your total grams per meal as far as this macronutrient is concerned.

No Wheat, No Rice

For best results during the Fat Wars 45-Day Transformation Plan, it is important to avoid wheat and rice of any kind. This means no bread, no pasta, and no rice for the duration of the nine weeks. These are the carbohydrate sources that seem to cause the greatest insulin spikes and cravings for sugar, so avoiding them will make things much easier. After the nine weeks, you can reintroduce them into your diet; the choice is yours.

Note: As mentioned in Chapter 11, "The Fat Wars Eating Principles," the final meal of the day (meal 5) should be adjusted to contain carbohydrates solely from fibrous vegetables, such as various forms of lettuce. Other fibrous, low-glycemic vegetables can be found in Chapter 6, listed in the low-glycemic vegetable column of the Fat Wars Glycemic Index. The reason for this adjustment in the evening is that it allows for effective fat burning through maximum growth-hormone release due to lowered insulin levels. Your last meal is the only meal that requires this adjustment.

PUTTING YOUR EXERCISE PLAN TOGETHER

The exercise portion of the transformation plan is key to your success, since exercising is how you will increase your body's ability to burn fat. I base my recommendations on the periodization philosophy of resistance training, which other trainers and I have used with great success for fat loss. The routines are progressively changed for maximized benefits. There are also two different programs of routines for you to do once you establish your exercise habit. The first one consists of three resistance-training sessions per week (on Monday, Wednesday, and Friday); each session includes routines that work muscles all over your body.

The second program is a split routine. It involves resistance training four times per week; in this program, you work two separate groups of muscles in your body, twice each week each, for a total of four training sessions. I highly recommend that you remain very active on the off days of the resistance portion of the program, including weekends.

When exercising, you should aim for a target heart rate that maximizes fat burning. The goal is to keep your system from running out of oxygen and switching to sugar for fuel instead of fat. Your target heart rate is 50% to 60% of (220 minus your age). As an example, if you are 40 years old, you would subtract 40 from 220 to get 180; 50% to 60% of 180 gives you a training intensity level of 90 to 108 beats per minute. You should start out at the lower number, in this case around 90 beats per minute, and increase to the high part of the range as you get in better shape.

Note: Please understand that it is not imperative to measure your target heart rate for success. A good indicator of effective fat burning is to make sure that you are able to carry on a conversation without huffing and puffing while you are exercising. As long as you are able to do this, you are transferring enough oxygen to the muscles for effective fat burning.

You can measure your heart rate a couple of different ways. One is manual, and the other requires a mechanical device that takes regular measurements of your pulse.

Manual Method: You can get a good pulse read at two areas on your body; one is on your wrist, and the other is on your neck.

- On the underside of your wrist, locate the tendon that runs from the forearm to the hand. Next, using the index and middle fingers of the opposite hand, press the thumb side of that tendon just below your hand. You should feel your radial pulse.
- You can also feel your pulse by locating your carotid artery (the main artery that supplies blood to the brain) on your neck. Place your index and middle fingers just below your jaw (on the same side as your hand). Feel around for a slight indentation and keep your fingers gently pressed on that spot until you feel your pulse.

Exercising Safely

Because *Fat Wars* is not intended to be an exercise manual, but instead is meant to offer a suggested exercise protocol to get you started on your successful fat-burning way, you should enlist the aid of a qualified personal trainer to ensure that you do the resistance exercises properly and safely (check out the Fat Wars Web site for a qualified Fat Wars trainer in your area). If you do not want to do this, or can't afford the services of a trainer, then I recommend that you purchase a book on resistance training that has easy-to-follow diagrams of each exercise, or visit the Fat Wars Web site, where you'll find pictures of exercises. One recommended title is *Weight Training for Dummies* by Suzanne Schlosberg and Liz Neporent.

If you have any physical limitations, joint pains, chronic muscle aches, or if you experience sudden or recurring dizziness at any time during your exercises, you must check with your health care provider before continuing. If you haven't been active for some time, it is advisable to check with your health care provider before you start.

- Once you have located your pulse in either spot, count the beats for 10 full seconds and multiply by 6 (one full minute). *Voilà,* that's your heart rate.

Mechanical Method: There are many heart-rate monitors available on the market that automatically measure your heart rate while you're exercising. If you can afford a quality device, it is a very practical tool for staying within your target heart rate. Some of the recommended brand names will be posted on the Fat Wars Web site at *www.fatwars.com.*

Week 1

Use this week to ease into your new lifestyle commitments. If you are not familiar with stretching movements, use this time to find a qualified fitness trainer who can take you through the routine until you can do them easily.

Monday through Friday, do the following:

Warm-up	5 minutes of slow walking
Resistance training	None
Aerobic	Take a 1-hour walk every day this week (preferably first thing in the morning on an empty stomach). When you are walking, be aware of your posture: Your chin should be held high and your back should be straight. Swing your arms. Get your whole body into the walk. There should be a good amount of deep breathing, but not so much that you are gasping for air—you should be able to carry on a conversation.
Abdominal crunches	3 sets of abdominal crunches on a stability ball following each walk. Start with sets of 5 repetitions (reps).
Cool down	Stretch for about 10 minutes.

Week 2

Add a routine of eight resistance exercises on Monday, Wednesday, and Friday of this week. Use dumbbells for all the exercises listed below in order to stimulate the best muscle contractions.

Follow the rep schemes presented here. If, for example, a specified rep scheme calls for 20 repetitions per set, it is important to the outcome of the set that you perform only that number of reps. You should be barely able to complete the final repetition. Carefully pick the weight that you are going to use. When you are able to do more than the recommended number of reps, increase the size of the weight.

Instructions for Proper Abdominal Crunches on a Stability Ball
Based on my experience and the experience of my colleagues in the fitness field, it is best to perform your crunches with a stability ball instead of on the floor. When performed on the floor, you do not utilize the abdominal muscles effectively due to the limited range of motion. By replacing floor crunches with crunches performed on the stability ball, you will not only avoid injury (if the exercises are performed correctly), but you will also greatly enhance the effectiveness of the exercise. Please visit *www.fatwars.com* for visuals of this exercise.

Fit yourself onto the correct-sized ball. If you're
- shorter than 5'3", choose a 45 cm ball
- 5'3" to 5'8", choose a 55 cm ball
- 5'9" to 6'0", choose a 65 cm ball
- 6'1" or taller, choose a 75 cm ball

When seated on the ball with your feet together, your knees and hips should both be at 90-degree angles.
- To begin an abdominal crunch on the ball, start from the seated position and lower your body slowly down by moving your feet away from the ball. As you are moving your feet away from the ball, progressively place more of your back on to the ball. When the ball is supported under your lower back, you are in your correct start position.
- From here, start the exercise by drawing your bellybutton toward your spine and extending backward until your shoulder blades and head rest on the ball (you are "wrapped" around the ball). Now slowly and steadily curl up from the head and upper torso, flexing forward until you reach a point near vertical. Slowly reverse the curl and return to the start position.
- While performing this exercise, keep your tongue on the roof of your mouth, behind your front teeth for proper anatomical alignment.

Cautions:
- Don't jerk yourself up to achieve this exercise. Perform it at a slow and steady pace.
- If you experience dizziness or nausea during this exercise, an underlying arterial condition in the spine may exist. Stop immediately and contact an orthopedic physical therapist for evaluation.

- Do not wear jewelry, watches, or belts when on the stability ball. They may inadvertently puncture the ball.
- Do not substitute abdominal machines or devices that you may see on TV or in a gym setting. They are highly dysfunctional and will often lead to lower-back injury.

Perform one set of 20 repetitions for each exercise, with a one-minute rest between sets.

Monday, Wednesday, and Friday

Warm-up	10 minutes of walking or riding a bike to increase the blood flow

Exercises

Resistance training	Sets	Repetitions
Dumbbell Squats (thighs)	1	20
Reverse (Step-Back) Lunge (rear of thigh)	1	20
Dumbbell Bench-Press (back)	1	20
Dumbbell Rows (back)	1	20
Dumbbell Side Laterals (shoulders)	1	20
Dumbbell Curls (biceps)	1	20
Dumbbell Tricep Extension (triceps)	1	20
Standing Calf Raises (calves)	1	20
Aerobic exercise	Walk for 30 minutes at your target heart rate. Warm up and cool down for about 5 minutes at a slower pace.	
Abdominal crunches	3 sets of abdominal crunches following each walk. Do 10 reps in each set.	
Cool down	About 10 minutes of stretching	

Tuesday and Thursday

Warm-up	5 minutes of slow walking
Resistance training	None
Aerobic exercise	30 to 60 minutes of walking
Abdominal crunches	3 sets of abdominal crunches following each walk. Do 10 reps in each set.
Cool down	About 10 minutes of stretching

Weeks 3 and 4

You will be staying with the same weight for both sets in your resistance-training program. Since your muscles will be fatiguing on each consecutive set, don't be surprised if you have trouble doing the 20 repetitions on the second set. Do as many as you can (try your best to get 20 reps).

Monday, Wednesday, and Friday

Warm-up	10 minutes of walking or riding a bike to increase the blood flow

Exercises

Resistance training	Sets	Repetitions
Dumbbell Squats (thighs)	2	20
Dumbbell Stiff-Reverse (Step-Back) Lunge (rear of thigh)	2	20
Dumbbell Bench-Press (chest)	2	20
Dumbbell Rows (back)	2	20
Dumbbell Side Laterals (shoulders)	2	20
Dumbbell Curls (biceps)	2	20
Dumbbell Tricep Extension (triceps)	2	20
Standing Calf Raises (calves)	2	20
Aerobic exercise	Walk for 30 minutes at your target heart rate. Warm up and cool down at a slower pace.	
Abdominal crunches	3 sets of abdominal crunches following each walk. Do 15 reps in each set.	
Cool down	About 10 minutes of stretching	

Tuesday and Thursday

Warm-up	5 minutes of slow walking
Resistance training	None
Aerobic exercise	30 to 60 minutes of walking
Abdominal crunches	3 sets of abdominal crunches following each walk. Do 15 reps in each set.
Cool down	Stretch for about 10 minutes.

Week 5

The number of sets per resistance training exercise will increase from two to three. The number of repetitions in each set will change from 20 to 15.

Monday and Friday workouts will be at full force, but on Wednesday, ease up on your training intensity (i.e., use a lighter weight), moving through each exercise with as little rest as possible (one minute at the most). Although the weights can be eased up a bit on Wednesday, the repetitions stay the same, allowing for an easier workout.

On each day, stay with the same weight for all three sets. Since your muscles will be fatiguing on each consecutive set, don't be surprised if you have trouble doing the 15 repetitions on the second and third set. Do as many as you can (try your best to get 15 reps).

Monday, Wednesday, and Friday

Warm-up	10 minutes of walking or riding a bike to increase the blood flow

Exercises

Resistance training	Sets	Repetitions
Dumbbell Squats (thighs)	3	15
Dumbbell Stiff-Legged Dead Lifts (rear of thigh)	3	15
Dumbbell Bench Press (chest)	3	15
Dumbbell Rows (back)	3	15
Dumbbell Side Laterals (shoulders)	3	15
Dumbbell Curls (biceps)	3	15
Dumbbell Tricep Extensions (triceps)	3	15
Standing Calf Raises (calves)	3	15
Aerobic exercise	Walk for 30 minutes at your target heart rate. Warm up and cool down at a slower pace.
Abdominal crunches	3 sets of abdominal crunches following each walk. Do 20 reps in each set.
Cool down	About 10 minutes of stretching

Tuesday and Thursday

Warm-up	5 minutes of slow walking
Resistance training	None
Aerobic exercise	30 to 60 minutes of walking
Abdominal crunches	3 sets of abdominal crunches following each walk. Do 20 reps in each set.
Cool down	About 10 minutes of stretching

Weeks 6 to 9

Now that your metabolism has been jump-started and your body has adapted to the weight training from the previous month, your workout format will change to the split routine. Instead of repeating the same training session to work all muscle groups, you will now use two different training sessions that target two different sets of muscle groups. This split routine will allow some muscle groups to gain extra rest (for recuperation) while others are being trained. During these weeks, you will train with weights on Monday and Tuesday and then again on Thursday and Friday.

You will now perform two exercises for each muscle group instead of one. Up until this point in your transformation program, you have been performing compound exercises, which are exercises that use a number of muscle groups. The split routines incorporate both a compound exercise and an isolation exercise. Unlike compound exercises, isolation exercises work only a single muscle or a specific group of muscles.

You will also add a barbell exercise to this part of your transformation routine. There are three sets in the first exercise for each muscle group, followed by two sets for the second exercise (the isolation exercise), for a total of five sets per body part. Certain smaller muscle groups (such as the muscles of the arms) will only require three sets of one exercise in total. The repetitions per exercise will be 10 to 12. This will allow for heavier weights than previously used for increased muscle strength, size, and function.

Follow this routine for the remainder of the nine weeks.

Monday and Friday

Warm-up	10 minutes of walking or riding a bike to increase the blood flow		
Exercises			
Resistance training		**Sets**	**Repetitions**
Barbell Squats (thighs)		3	10 to 12
Seated Leg Extensions		2	10 to 12
Stiff-Legged Dead Lift (rear of thigh)		3	10 to 12
Lying Leg Curls		2	10 to 12
Side Laterals (shoulders)		3	10 to 12
Calf Raises (calves)		3	10 to 12
Aerobic exercise	Walk for 20 minutes at your target heart rate. Warm up and cool down at a slower pace.		
Abdominal crunches	3 sets of abdominal crunches following each walk. Do 25 reps in each set.		
Cool down	About 10 minutes of stretching		

Tuesday and Thursday

Warm-up	10 minutes of walking or riding a bike to increase the blood flow

Exercises

Resistance training	Sets	Repetitions
Bench Press	3	10 to 12
Incline Press	2	10 to 12
Bent-Over Rows	3	10 to 12
Seated Cable Rows	2	10 to 12
Standing Barbell Curls (biceps)	3	10 to 12
Barbell Tricep Extension (triceps)	3	10 to 12
Aerobic exercise	Walk for 20 minutes at your target heart rate. Warm up and cool down at a slower pace.	
Abdominal crunches	3 sets of abdominal crunches following each walk. Do 25 reps per set.	
Cool down	About 10 minutes of stretching	

Wednesday

Warm-up	5 minutes of slow walking
Resistance training	None
Aerobic exercise	30 to 60 minutes of walking
Abdominal crunches	3 sets of abdominal crunches following each walk. Do 25 reps in each set.
Cool down	About 10 minutes of stretching

After the 45-Day Transformation Period

If you stick with the advice in this section, you will be successful in achieving your Fat Wars goal. Once the 45-day transformation period is over, your new life will be just beginning. All the workout suggestions have been based on a scientific approach to progressive resistance using a periodization training philosophy. The periodization philosophy allows for three four-month cycles of various training routines to be performed in any given year. This type of training allows for constant improvement in all areas of athleticism.

Periodization Training

Periodization training is any training plan that changes your workouts at regular intervals. It involves changing many variables pertaining to a workout routine, including the number of repetitions in a set, the kind of exercises performed, the amount of weight used, and the amount of time allowed for rest in between your sets. It is a scientifically sound way to ensure continual improvements and not hit the all-too-common training plateau, where at a certain time in a person's training cycle, all progress seems to come to an abrupt halt.

Periodization training includes cycles of intense and less intense training periods throughout the year so that you reduce long intervals of stress on your body. When people train the conventional way, they sometimes accumulate stress to the point of doing damage. By alternating intense and less intense workout cycles, muscle strain and training plateaus are prevented. A typical periodization plan will consist of three four-month cycles. Each month would allow for a new set of training rules, for instance:

- The first month may call for a high-rep scheme of 20 reps per set, but only one or two sets per exercise. Therefore, you would be lifting relatively light weights (low intensity).
- The second month may consist of a lower rep scheme of 12 to 15 reps per set with perhaps two to three sets per exercise, allowing you to lift slightly heavier weights (higher intensity).
- The third month would call for a still lower rep scheme of 8 to 10 reps per set and three to four sets per exercise, allowing for relatively heavy weights to increase strength and size (intense).
- The final month (month 4) would be the most intense, using the lowest rep scheme of four to six reps per set and three to five sets per exercise, allowing for the heaviest weights used in the four months, which would further increase the strength of the muscle fibers.

After the fourth month of training, you would begin the routine again at the first month to allow for maximum recovery and recuperation from the most intense month of the routine. There are three of these cycles in a typical year. Of course, this is just a very generalized outlook on the principles of periodization training, but it's enough to give you some insight into periodization's principles. For a detailed approach to this training method, you should read *Periodization Breakthrough* by Steven Fleck and Dr. William Kraemer.

The routines presented in the Fat Wars 45-Day Transformation Plan will bring you through two of these four-week-long periodization cycles. The goal of this transformation plan is an increase in muscle size and fat-burning activity. The basic periodization goal per cycle is to progress from high-volume (higher reps/sets), low-intensity (lighter weights) training through the first two cycles to low-volume (lower reps/sets) and high-intensity (heavier weights) training through the final two cycles. As you continue on your new life path (and I know you will), you should complete the last two cycles of a properly designed training program by progressively lowering the repetitions of the exercises performed while increasing the weights used. Please refer to a well-designed training manual or get help from a qualified personal trainer versed in periodization training. Cardio activity should remain constant throughout the various cycles. This way your body will continue to progress and avoid any plateaus.

THE FIVE KEYS TO REACHING YOUR FAT-LOSS GOALS

1: Visualize

In order to achieve, you must really believe, and in order to believe, you must first visualize yourself attaining the goal.

- Be as detailed as possible when you visualize. Picture yourself in your new body and enjoying your new lifestyle. How do you look in your new body? What do you feel like? How are people around you responding? How confident do you feel? How energized are you? Whatever you really want to look like, picture it as if it has already happened.
- Take a picture of yourself wearing a bathing suit. Place it where you will be able to see it often. Nothing motivates people more than being reminded of how they looked before they started. Whenever you feel like going off your plan, look at the picture and visualize your new body.
- Believe. In a sense, it's like acting; you need to play the part of the person you want to become. No matter what happens between now and the day you hope to achieve your goal, in your mind you have already achieved it. You have already accepted the reality of the new you.

2: Write Down Your Fat-Loss Goal

Be specific, but also be realistic about the time frame for achieving your goal. For instance, if you presently register 40% body fat but your goal is to be at 24%, don't expect to reach your goal in a month. (Note that you're not setting a target for weight loss in pounds—the leaner you will be adding fat-burning muscle.) Be honest with yourself—don't set yourself up for fail-ure. Write down achievable timelines for your objective: the first three weeks, the second three weeks, and beyond. Your goal for the first three weeks could be to get your new routines in place; by six weeks you could aim to lose 3% to 4% body fat. Be specific with dates. Don't just write "in three weeks." Write down the actual date three, six, and nine weeks from when you start.

Identify why you've set your goals; for instance, "I want to lose 3% to 4% body fat by November 30 because I'm going to Hawaii and I want to look good. I also want to lose this fat because I know that I will feel better about myself and have more energy to enjoy my trip. Once I feel better, I will continue to work toward the healthy state I always knew I could achieve. My health is really what matters most to me. Losing this weight is only the beginning of a whole new me." Be as specific as possible.

After you've told yourself what you're doing and why, let others know what you are doing. You must be sincere about this step: If you jokingly say, "You won't recognize me next summer," then you won't take it seriously. Be strong in your conviction. Trust me, there's no better way to guarantee suc-cess than putting extra pressure on yourself by letting your friends know what you are striving for. Don't be afraid to ask for their support. Believe me, they will be the first to let you know if you're not sticking to your plan.

3: Write Down What You Need to Change

In order to follow the Fat Wars 45-Day Transformation Plan, you will have to make some changes. Let's be realistic here. You have developed—how shall we say it?—some bad habits along the way that got you where you are today. Many of them have to go. How about starting with those late nights that deprive you of badly needed sleep? That one positive change will mean that you will be able to wake up one hour earlier each day, and you'll have time to complete the energizing exercise portion of the plan.

You will also have to assess what you've been eating. Plan the changes that will help you burn fat, and eliminate much of what you've come to rely on as comfort foods. Write down everything you can think of that you need to change to guarantee success. If you've never tried anything like this before, the changes will feel dramatic—but the emerging new you is worth it. If you've tried lots of diets before and you've been exercising, it will be a matter of making adjustments. Remember that after 45 days, you'll feel so great that no one will have to convince you to continue.

4: Keep a Log of Your Progress

It's time to take charge of your success. Remove all the guesswork and chaos from your training and diet program by keeping an accurate record of each workout and each day's food intake. Winning your personal Fat War requires careful planning and organization, setting priorities, and being willing to spend some time tracking your changes (or lack of them).

If you are willing to keep a log of your training and diet activities, then you will have a precise record of what works best for you and how much you've really changed. Make a training journal by noting what you did to warm up and cool down, what resistance exercises you did at what weights and with how many repetitions, what aerobic exercises you did and how many stomach crunches, and any comments/thoughts. A training journal will help you:

- see progress from each workout;
- know how many repetitions you performed and how much weight you used in your last workout;
- have an accurate record of the exercises or routines that did and didn't work for you;
- know when to make adjustments in your training cycles.

A diet journal will help you:

- keep track of how many calories you are taking in;
- keep an accurate record of the best calorie intake for your needs;
- ensure that you are within your proper macronutrient profile;
- know when to make adjustments in your food intake.

5: Take Responsibility for Reaching Your Goal, but Be Patient with Yourself

Don't sweat it if you lose a battle or two. None of us is perfect. Most of us work long hours and have commitments that can get in the way of following the Fat Wars plan perfectly. The key is to keep your eye on the big picture, which is permanent fat loss. If you slip up now and then, it won't make a big difference in the scheme of things.

Remember that changing a lifetime of bad habits—or even making minor adjustments—is not something that you can do overnight. But as the story of the rock and the sand showed, if you add one grain of sand a day, eventually the rock will move. If you aren't seeing the results you are looking for in the (reasonable) time frames you have given yourself, take a hard look at your logbooks. Are you doing everything it takes to accomplish your goal? Can you take your efforts to a new level now that you've made a start? Remember that if you take in too many calories in any form, the excess will be deposited in your fat account. If you rarely take your fat-burning engine out for a spin, that stored fuel is going to stay in storage. Do everything in your power to stay on track. Think of yourself standing in front of that full-length mirror looking at your new body, and think of yourself enjoying each day with energy to spare. How will that feel?

Congratulations! You are well on your way to a new, healthier, happier, leaner you. So what are you waiting for? Get your battle strategy together. It's time to win the Fat Wars!

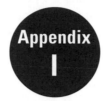

Fat Wars Product Supplement

Recommendations

Throughout the book there have been recommendations for supplements and other products. Below you will find some more specific suggestions. Some of these products are marketed by ehn Inc., which also represents the award-winning greens+ in Canada. I have confidently recommended these products for a number of years, believing them to be among the best in the industry. Early last year I agreed to come aboard the greens+ team and develop cutting-edge products for the company, some of which are transform+, proteins+, lean+, crave-free, protect, enact+, and A.G.E. inhibitors. I have no other affiliation with any other manufacturer at this time.

Through my many years in the health industry I have come to realize that there are only a handful of respectable and trustworthy product manufacturers. The recommendations I have presented here are, to the best of my knowledge, some of the top ones in the industry.

Note: All the recommended supplements in this section (unless specified as available only in the U.S.) can be found at your local health food retailer.

Whey Protein Isolate (proteins+ and transform+)

AlphaPure® is produced using a patented isolation process for whey protein isolate, creating the highest biological value of any protein on the market today. AlphaPure® contains 2.5 times the cysteine levels present in other whey protein isolates. AlphaPure® provides an excellent and unsurpassed source of natural glutathione builders.

The levels of the amino acid tryptophan in AlphaPure® are triple that of other whey protein isolates. Tryptophan is needed by the body to produce the neurotransmitter serotonin. Through extensive research over the past 40 years it has been established that the activity level of serotonin has a material impact on levels of insomnia, pain sensitivity, anxiety, and depression. Serotonin has also been demonstrated to have appetite suppressant qualities.

AlphaPure® contains the highest levels of glycomacropeptides (GMPs) found in any whey protein product. GMPs are powerful stimulators of a hormone called cholecystokinin (CCK), which plays many essential roles in our gastrointestinal system. CCK stimulates the release of enzymes from the pancreas and increases gall bladder contraction and bowel motility. One of CCK's most incredible actions lies in its ability to regulate our food intake by sending satiation signals to the brain, making it a potential diet aid. In animal studies, a rise in CCK is always followed by a large reduction in food intake. In human studies, whey protein glycomacropeptides were shown to increase CCK production by 415% within 20 minutes after ingestion.

AlphaPure® is a registered trademark of:

Protein Fractionations Inc.
1146 Castlefield Ave
Toronto, Ontario, M6B 1E9
Tel: 416-783-8315
Fax: 416-783-7589
AlphaPure® is carried exclusively in Canada by ehn. Inc.

ehn Inc. (Greens+ Canada)
317 Adelaide Street West, Suite 501
Toronto, Ontario, M5V 1P9
Tel: 416-977-3505
Toll-free: 877-500-7888
Fax: 416-977-4184
Web Site: *www.greenspluscanada.com*

Soy Protein Isolate

Look for the Supro® non-GMO brand of soy protein isolate. Supro® non-GMO brand of soy protein isolate contains the highest quality water-extracted soy protein on the market today. Supro® non-GMO soy protein isolate has a biological value of 100, the same as an egg when it comes to protein quality. The product transform+ only uses non-GMO soy protein isolate as its soy protein source.

Supro® is a registered trademark of:
Protein Technologies International
P.O. Box 88940
St. Louis, Missouri 63188
Toll-free: Consumer Inquiries: 877-SOY4HEALTH (877-769-4432)
        Customer or Business Inquiries: 800-325-7108
Fax: 314-982-2461

Essential Fatty Acid (EFA) Manufacturers and Distributors

Omega Balance Oil and Flax Oil

Omega Nutrition Canada Inc.
1924 Franklin Street
Vancouver, British Columbia, V5L 1R2
Tel: 604-253-4677
Toll-free: 800-661-3529
Fax: 604-253-4893
Web Site: *www.omegaflo.com*

Udo's Choice Oil and Flax Oil

Flora Distributors Ltd.
7400 Fraser Park Drive
Burnaby, British Columbia, V5J 5B9
Toll-free: 800-663-0617
Fax: 606-436-6060
Web Site: *www.florahealth.com*

Bioriginal Oils

Bioriginal Food & Science Corp.
102 Melville Street
Saskatoon, Saskatchewan, S7J 0R1
Tel: 306-975-9268
Fax: 306-242-3829

Fish Oils, EPA, and DHA
Ocean Nutrition Canada Ltd.
747 Bedford Highway
Bedford, Nova Scotia, V4A 2Z7
Tel: 902-457-2399
Toll-free: 800-980-8889
Fax: 902-457-2357
Web Site: *www.ocean-nutrition.com*

Evening Primrose Oil (GLA)
Efamol Canada (1998) Ltd.
Scotia Centre
35 Webster Street
Kentville, Nova Scotia, B4N 1H4
Toll-free: 800-539-3326
Fax: 902-678-2885
Web Site: *www.efamol.com*

Flora Distributors Ltd.
7400 Fraser Park Drive
Burnaby, British Columbia, V5J 5B9
Toll-free: 800-663-0617
Fax: 606-436-6060
Web Site: *www.florahealth.com*

Purity Professionals (professional distributor)
Division of Purity Life Health products
2975 Lake City Way
Burnaby, British Columbia, V5A 2Z6
Toll-free: 888-443-3323
Fax: 888-223-6111
E-mail: professional@puritylife.com

According to research presented in the *New England Journal of Medicine* (June 13, 1996), enteric-coated fish oils may present an enhanced method of delivery, especially in people with compromised gastrointestinal systems.

Concentrated Green Foods
Not all concentrated green foods are the same quality. Look for powders that contain an array of natural organic greens and herbs. I highly recommend the multi award-winning greens+ formula. *Note:* There is a full serving of greens+ in every serving of the gold medal-winning transform+ formula listed above.

ehn Inc. (Greens+ Canada)
317 Adelaide Street West, Suite 501
Toronto, Ontario, M5V 1P9
Tel: 416-977-3505
Toll-free: 877-500-7888
Fax: 416-977-4184
Web Site: *www.greenspluscanada.com*

Anti-Craving Formula (crave-free)

Many people cannot fight their physiological urge to binge eat, especially where insulin-spiking carbohydrates are concerned. It is important to recognize that in many cases the failure to lose your excess fat may largely be due to various biochemical imbalances in brain chemicals that quite literally drive you to eat excessively. It is sometimes almost impossible to ignore the insatiable craving for these foods, and when we finally give in we feel a great wave of relief that unfortunately lasts only a little while and leaves us with another pound or two.

In Chapters 4, 9, and 12, I covered the various aspects of these brain chemicals (neurotransmitters) and how they affect the craving and award centers of your brain. One of the most important of these craving chemicals is serotonin. In Chapter 12, I dove a little deeper into the realm of cravings and how certain nutrients have been shown to help overcome insatiable cravings by modulating these brain chemicals (mostly serotonin). The various nutrients discussed in Chapter 12 have now been placed for your convenience into one formula called crave-free.

crave-free contains the following ingredients in effective ratios for continual craving reductions:

- *Griffonia* – (natural source of 5-hydroxytryptophan [5-HTP]) Can help to boost serotonin levels, reduce food cravings, and promote weight loss.
- *Rhodiola rosea* – Can help to decrease food intake by helping to increase the levels of the neurotransmitter dopamine.
- *Glutamine* – Is effective in decreasing cravings and addictive behavior.
- *Rhubarb root* – Has been shown in studies to be as effective as the one-time anti-craving drug fenfluramine, but importantly without the side effects.
- *Magnesium citrate* – Can help reduce cravings, particularly sugar and chocolate cravings in premenstrual women.
- *Chromium citrate* – Can help to prevent cravings for carbohydrates by regulation of blood sugar and normal insulin response.
- *Vitamin C* – Is required for the synthesis of neurotransmitters, including serotonin.

- *Pyridoxal-5-Phosphate* – (the active form of vitamin B6). Can regulate cravings by increasing levels of both serotonin and dopamine (through a process called decarboxylation).

WARNING: Those taking selective serotonin reuptake inhibitors, tricyclic anti-depressants, or monoamine oxidase inhibitors should consult a health care professional before taking this product.

crave-free is available exclusively through:
ehn Inc. (Greens+ Canada)
317 Adelaide Street West, Suite 501
Toronto, Ontario, M5V 1P9
Tel: 416-977-3505
Toll-free: 877-500-7888
Fax: 416-977-4184
Web Site: *www.greenspluscanada.com*

Network Antioxidant Formula (protect)

protect is a synergistic antioxidant formula containing the network antioxidants as discussed in Chapter 12. The formula is packed with antioxidant protection like no other formula on the market. protect contains: vitamins C and E (with mixed tocopherols), beta carotene (pro-vitamin A with mixed carotenoids), alpha lipoic acid, and CoQ10, along with grape seed extract, citrus bioflavanoids, European bilberry, lycopene, N-acetyl cysteine (NAC), and selenium.

Note: The best way to boost glutathione levels in the body is to take lipoic acid, NAC (or AlphaPure® protein found in proteins+ and transform+).

protect is available exclusively through:
ehn Inc. (Greens+ Canada)
317 Adelaide Street West, Suite 501
Toronto, Ontario, M5V 1P9
Tel: 416-977-3505
Toll-free: 877-500-7888
Fax: 416-977-4184
Web Site: *www.greenspluscanada.com*

Milk Thistle

Generally, milk thistle extracts come standardized to contain a minimum of 75% silymarin. At this potency, a dose of 50–100 milligrams two to three times daily will really boost liver cell activity and keep your fat-burning army marching along toward victory. One of the most effective formulas for liver function presently on the market is called liv-tone, marketed in Canada by:

ehn Inc. (Greens+ Canada)
317 Adelaide Street West, Suite 501
Toronto, Ontario, M5V 1P9
Tel: 416-977-3505
Toll-free: 877-500-7888
Fax: 416-977-4184
Web Site: *www.greenspluscanada.com*

Colostrum

As discussed in Chapter 12, colostrum is the pre-milk substance that is produced by the mother's mammary glands for only the first 24–48 hours after giving birth. It is important to state, however, that the earlier the colostrum is taken from the source the more potent it is. Studies show that colostrum harvested 12 hours after birth only contains one-third of the immune and growth factors present at birth.

This incredible substance, containing some of the most important immune and growth factors in cows, is identical in molecular formation to human colostrum and is therefore easily transferable from one species (cow) to another (human). For maximum potency and bioactivity, look for the following: The colostrum should be harvested from select Grade A dairy cows within the first six hours, and should be processed in a certified GMP facility under the strictest of quality standards using very low heat.

Carnitine

L-carnitine is a very powerful ally on your side in the Fat Wars. As mentioned, carnitine helps to transport fatty acids into the furnaces (mitochondria) of our cells so that it can be incinerated. L-carnitine is presently restricted in Canada; however, it is concentrated in colostrum, and supplementing with bovine colostrum may be a great way to increase natural carnitine levels.

Sequel Naturals Colostrum is distributed in Canada by:
Sequel Naturals
Toll free: 1-866-839-8863
E-mail: info@seqeulnaturals.com
Web Site: *www.sequelnaturals.com*

Pharmaceutical Grade L-Carnitine and Acetyl L-Carnitine
Available only in the United States:
Twin Laboratories Inc.
2120 Smithtown Avenue
Ronkonkoma, New York, 11779
Tel: 631-467-3140

Fax: 631-630-3486
Web Site: *www.twinlab.com*

Life Extension Foundation (mail order only)
995 South West 24th Street
Fort Lauderdale, Florida, 33315
Tel: 954-766-8433
Toll-free: 800-841-5433
Fax: 954-921-2069
Web Site: *www.lef.org*

lean+: The Ultimate Fat Wars Nutrient Formula

While there are a number of fat-burning nutrients listed individually, you don't have to hunt each of them down. Many can be found in combination with other fat-burning nutrients in a special formula available as lean+. Designed by author/researcher Brad King, it contains seven of the star players in the war on fat: *Citrus aurantium* (Bitter Orange or *zhi shi*); hydroxycitric acid (HCA); *Coleus forskohlii* extract; guggulipid; green tea extract; alpha-lipoic acid, and cayenne. Many of these were introduced in Chapter 12.

lean+ is a unique formula that targets a variety of biochemical problems inherent to weight loss, including the activation of the enzymes and messengers necessary for fat loss to occur.

lean+:

- increases the breakdown of stored fat (lipolysis) by activating fat-releasing enzymes and increasing intracellular communication;
- increases the metabolic rate through increased thermogenesis (body heat production) and stimulation of the thyroid;
- curbs excess appetite;
- improves the metabolism of carbohydrates (sugars) so fewer will convert to fat;
- inhibits the production of fat by the fat cells;
- increases energy;
- lowers LDL and VLDL ("bad") cholesterol levels while increasing HDL ("good") cholesterol levels;
- protects against damage by free radicals.

Ingredient Highlights:

- *Alpha-lipoic acid* is not only a potent antioxidant that helps to protect virtually all the tissues of the body, but also a cofactor for some of the key enzymes (alpha keto acid dehydrogenases) involved in generating energy from food and oxygen in mitochondria. Alpha-lipoic acid also helps to control excess sugar levels by improving carbohydrate metabolism and ensuring that fewer carbohydrates (sugars) are converted into fat. This improves energy levels as the metabolized carbohydrates become energy for your mind and body.

- *Cayenne* stimulates the production of ATP (fuel), thus increasing thermogenesis and stimulating the BAT cells so that more calories can be burned. It also aids in the absorption of the other ingredients.

- *Citrus aurantium* increases the breakdown of stored fat (lipolysis) by increasing the activity of the BAT cells and thus of thermogenesis and the metabolic rate. Unlike ephedra (Ma huang), caffeine or guarana, *Citrus aurantium* works by attaching its amines to the beta-3 (thermogenic receptor) receptor sites on a cell's surface without stimulating the central nervous system, and thus has none of the associated side effects or health risks.

- *Coleus forskohlii* increases the breakdown of stored fat (lipolysis) through the increase of the cellular messenger cAMP (cyclic adenosine monophosphate) in cells.

- *Grapefruit juice powder*—for those who remember the popular grapefruit diet of the '70s, here is the reason it worked. Grapefruit contains pectin, which helps to lower fat absorption and suppress the appetite. In lean+, the grapefruit juice powder complements the *Citrus aurantium* for increased efficacy.

- *Green tea* regulates the appetite and increases the activity of BAT cells, thus increasing thermogenesis and the burning of excess fat and calories. Green tea may also lower fat absorption by the intestines, and inhibit excess carbohydrates from being absorbed (inactivates amylase activity).

- *Guggulipid* contains plant compounds called guggulsterones that have been proven to regulate the metabolism by stimulating thyroid output. They help to convert inactive thyroid hormones into metabolically active ones (T4–T3), thus stimulating the BAT cells to increase thermogenesis and burn stored fat. Guggulipid also lowers the risk of coronary artery disease and "bad" cholesterol (LDL and VLDL) levels—both commonly associated with obesity.

- *Hydroxycitric acid (HCA)* from *Garcinia cambogia* curbs the appetite, inhibits the conversion of carbohydrates (sugars) into fat, reduces fat production and storage, and improves the rate of fat burning in cells by inhibiting an enzyme that blocks fat from being burned (malonyl CoA).

lean+ is available exclusively through:
ehn Inc. (Greens+ Canada)
317 Adelaide Street West, Suite 501
Toronto, Ontario, M5V 1P9
Tel: 416-977-3505
Toll-free: 877-500-7888
Fax: 416-977-4184
Web Site: *www.greenspluscanada.com*

Dr. Seaton's Advanced Hygiene System (see Chapter 2) High Performance Hygiene
24000 Mercantile Road, Suite 7
Cleveland, Ohio, 44122
Tel/Toll-free: 888-262-5700
Fax/Toll-free: 888-247-8500
Web Site: *www.advancedhealth.cc*

HGH Secretagogues
As mentioned in Chapter 2, naturally elevating levels of HGH through amino acid secretagogues is a great way to gain an upper hand in the Fat Wars. The one product I have reviewed that seems to contain all the amino acids necessary for effective HGH stimulation is the product SomaLife gHP by Soma Health Products Inc. You can contact the company toll-free at 1-877-769-4868.

Bio-DIM Supplements
Absorbable diindolylmethane supplements (Bio-DIM®) and information on healthy estrogen metabolism are available from:

ehn Inc. (greens+ Canada)
317 Adelaide Street West, Suite 501
Toronto, Ontario, M5V 1P9
Tel: 416-977-3505
Toll-free: 877-500-7888
Fax: 416-977-4184
Web Site: *www.greenspluscanada.com*

Note: Look for updated information on products, exercises, and research on the Fat Wars Web site at *www.fatwars.com.*

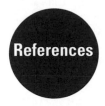

References

CHAPTER 1

Astrup, A., et al. "Pharmacology of Thermogenic Drugs," *Am J Clin Nutr*, 1992.

Barenys, M., et al. "Effect of Exercise and Protein Intake on Energy Expenditure in Adolescents," *Rev Esp Fisiol*, Dec, 1993, 49:4, 209-17.

Barnes, B.O. and L. Galton. *Hypothyroidism: The Unsuspected Illness*. New York: Harper & Row, 1976.

Berry, M., et al. "The Contribution of Hepatic Metabolism to Diet-Induced Thermogenesis," *Metabolism*, 1985, 34: 141-147.

Bornstein, S.R., et al. "Immunohistochemical and Ultrastructural Localization of Leptin and Leptin Receptor in Human White Adipose Tissue and Differentiating Human Adipose Cells in Primary Culture," *Diabetes*, 2000, 49: 4, 532-8.

Brent, G.A. "The Molecular Basis of Thyroid Action," *N Engl J Med*, 1994, 331: 847-853.

Chen, M.D., et al. "Zinc May Be a Mediator of Leptin Production in Humans," *Life Sci*, 2000, 66: 22, 2143-9.

Collins, S., et al. "Strain Specific Response to Beta-3 Adrenergic Receptor Agonist Treatment of Diet Induced Obesity in Mice," *Endocrinol*, 1997, 138: 405-413.

Dulloo, A.G. and D.S. Miller. "The Thermogenic Properties of Ephedrine/methylxanthine Mixtures: Human Studies," *Int J Obesity*, 1986 10: 467-81.

Fleury, C., et al. "Uncoupling Protein-2: A Novel Gene Linked to Obesity and Hyperinsulinemia," *Nat Genetics*, 1997, 15: 269-272.

Friedman, J.M. "Obesity in the New Millennium," *Nature*, 2000, 404: 6778, 632-4.

Ghorbam, M., et al. "Hypertrophy of Brown Adipocytes in Brown and White Adipose Tissues and Reversal of Diet Induced Obesity in Rats Treated with a Beta-3 Adrenoceptor Agonist," *Biochem Pharmacol*, 1997, 54: 121-131.

Goldberg, S. *Clinical Biochemistry Made Ridiculously Simple*, Edition 2, MedMaster, Inc., Miami, FL, 1997.

Gura, T. "Uncoupling Proteins Provide New Clue to Obesity's Causes," *Science*, May 29, 1998, 280: 1369-1370.

Harper, M.E. "Obesity Research Continues to Spring Leaks," *Clin Invest Med*, Aug, 20: 239-44.

James, W.P.T. and P. Trayhum. "Thermogenesis and Obesity," *British Med Bulletin*, 1981, 37(1): 43-48.

Kaats, G. "Effects of Multiple Herbal Formulation on Body Composition, Blood, Chemistry, Vital Signs and Self-Reported Energy Levels and Appetite Control," *Int J Obesity*, 1994.

King, B.J. and M.A. Schmidt. *Bio-Age: Ten Steps to A Younger You*, Macmillan Canada, 2001.

Kopecky, J. "Mitochondrial Energy Metabolism, Uncoupling Proteins and Adipose Tissue
      Accumulation," *Sb Lek*, 1998, 99 (3): 219-25.

Mersmann, H. "Evidence of Classic Beta-3 Adrenergic Receptors in Porcine Adipocytes,"
      J Anim Sci, May, 1996, 74:5: 984-92.

Orban, Z., et al. "The Interaction between Leptin and the Hypothalamic-Pituitary-Thyroid
      Axis," *Hormone Metabolic Research*, 30: 231-35, 1998.

Ricquier, D. "Uncoupling Protein-2 (UCP2): Molecular and Genetic Studies," *Int J Obes Relat
      Metab Disord*, Jun, 1999, 23 Suppl 6: S38-42.

Salas, S.J. "Influence of Adiposity on the Thermic Effect of Food and Exercise in Lean and
      Obese Adolescents," *Int J Obes Relat Metab Disord*, Dec 17, 1993, 12: 717-22.

Schmidt, M.A. *Smart Fats*, Frog, Ltd., 1997.

Schrauwen, P., et al. "Skeletal Muscle UCP2 and UCP3 Expression in Trained and Untrained
      Male Subjects," *Int J Obes Relat Metab Disord*, Sep 1999 (9): 966-72.

Schrauwen P., et al. "Human Uncoupling Proteins and Obesity," *Obes Res*, Jan 1999, 7(1):
      97-105.

Sears, B. *The Anti-Aging Zone*, New York: HarperCollins, Inc., 1999.

Soukas, A., et al. "Leptin-Specific Patterns of Gene Expression in White Adipose Tissue,"
      Genes Dev, 14: 8, 963-80, 2000.

Yang, Y., et al. "Multiple Actions of Beta Adrenergic Agonists on Skeletal Muscle and Adipose
      Tissue," *Biochem J*, 1989.

CHAPTER 2

Aiello, L.C. and P. Wheeler. "The Expensive-Tissue Hypothesis: The Brain and the Digestive
      System in Human and Primate Evolution," *Current Anthropology*, 1995, 36 (2): 199-221.

Atkins, R. *Dr. Atkins' New Diet Revolution*, New York: M. Evans & Co., 1999.

Cassidy, C.M. "Nutrition and Health in Agriculturists and Hunter-Gatherers: A Case Study of
      Two Prehistoric Populations," *Nutritional Anthropology*, Pleasantville, New York: 117-145.

Challem, J., et al. *Syndrome X: The Complete Nutritional Program to Prevent and Reverse Insulin
      Resistance*, New York: John Wiley & Sons, 2001.

Crist, D.M., et al. "Body Composition Response to Exogenous GH during Training in
      Highly Conditioned Adults," *J Appl Physiol*, Aug 1988, 65:2: 579-84.

Curtis, H. *Biology*, 4th ed. New York: Worth Publishers, 1986.

Dilman, V.M. *The Grand Biological Clock*, Moscow: Mir, 1989.

Eades, M.R., and M.D. Eades. *Protein Power*, New York: Bantam Books, 1999.

Eaton, S.B, et al. "An Evolutionary Perspective Enhances Understanding of Human
      Nutritional Requirements," *J of Nutr*, June 1996, 126: 1732-40.

Eaton, S.B. "Humans, Lipids and Evolution," *Lipids*, 1992, 27(10): 814-820.

Galbo, H. "Endocrinology and Metabolism in Exercise," *Int J Sports Med*, 1981, 2:125.

Goldwasser P. and J. Feldman. "Association of Serum Albumin and Mortality Risk,"
      J Clin Epidemiol, 1997, 50: 693-703.

Graci, S. *The Food Connection*, Toronto: Macmillan Canada, 2001.

Guezennec, C.Y. "Role of Lipids on Endurance Capacity in Man," *Int J Sports Med*, 1992,
      13(suppl 1): S114-S118.

Heleniak, E. and B. Aston. "Prostaglandins, Brown Fat and Weight Loss," *Med Hypoth*, 1989,
      28:13-3.

Klatz, R. and C. Kahn. *Grow Young with HGH*, New York: HarperCollins, 1997.

Patterson, C.R. *Essentials of Biochemistry*, London: Pittman Books, 1983, 38.

Peters, T. *All about Albumin*, San Diego: Academic Press, 1996.

Rudman, D., et al. "Effects of Human Growth Hormone in Men over 60 Years Old," *NE J Med*, 323: 1-6, 1990.

Samra, J.S., et al. "Suppression of the Nocturnal Rise in Growth Hormone Reduces Subsequent Lipolysis in Subcutaneous Adipose Tissue," *Eur J Clin Invest*, 1999, 29 (12): 1045-52.

Scheen, A.J. "From Obesity to Diabetes: Why, When and Who?" *Acta Clin Belg*, 2000, 55: 1, 9-15.

Seaton, K. "Carrying Capacity of Blood in Aging." Presented at the Anti-Aging conference, Las Vegas, 1999. Abstract available from Advanced Health Products, LLC, Beachwood, Ohio. Ph: 1-888-262-5700.

Sonntag, W., et al. "Moderate Caloric Restriction Alters the Subcellular Distribution of Somatostatin mRNA and Increases Growth Hormone Pulse Amplitude in Aged Animals," *Neuroendocrinology*, May, 1995, 61:5: 601-8.

Sonntag, W.E., et al. "Pleiotropic Effects of Growth Hormone and Insulin-like Growth Factor (IGF)-1 on Biological Aging: Inferences from Moderate Caloric-restricted Animals," *J Gerontol A Biol Sci Med Sci*, Dec. 1999, 54:12: B521-38.

Taskinen, M.R. and E. Nikkila. "Lipoprotein Lipase Of Adipose Tissue & Skeletal Muscle In Human Obesity," *Metabolism*, 1981, 30:810-17.

Xu, X. and W.E. Sonntag. "Moderate Caloric Restriction Prevents the Age-related Decline in Growth Hormone Receptor Signal Transduction," *J Gerontol A Biol Sci Med Sci*, Mar, 1996, 51:2: B167-74.

Yamashita, S. and S. Melmed. "Effects of Insulin on Rat Pituitary Cells: Inhibition of Growth Hormone Secretion and MRNA Levels," *Diabetes*, 1986, 35:440:447.

Yudkin, J. "Evolutionary and Historical Changes in Dietary Carbohydrates," *Amer J Clin Nutr*, 1967, 20(2): 108-115.

CHAPTER 3

Barnhart, Edward R. *Physicians' Desk Reference*, 45th ed, Oradell, NJ: Medical Economics Co., 1991.

Bhasin, S., et al. "The Effects of Supraphysiologic Doses of Testosterone on Muscle Size and Strength in Normal Men," *New Engl J Med*, July 1996, 335, no. 1: 1-7.

Campbell, D.R. and M.S. Kurzer. "Flavonoid Inhibition of Aromatase Enzyme Activity in Human Preadipocytes," *J Steroid Biochem Mol Biol*, Sept 1993, 46, no. 3: 381-8.

Fisher, B., et al. "Strength Training Parameters in the Edmonton Police Force Following Supplementation with Elk Velvet Antler (EVA)," 1998.

Hryb, D.J., et al. "The Effect of Extracts of the Roots of the Stinging Nettle (Urtica dioica) on the Interaction of SHBG with Its Receptor on Human Prostatic Membranes," *Planta Med* 61, no. 1 (February 1995): 31-2.

Hsieh, C., and J. Granstrom. "Staying Young Forever: Putting New Research Findings into Practice," *Life Extension* (December 1999).

_____ et al. "Predictors of Sex Hormone Levels Among the Elderly: A Study in Greece," *J of Clin Endocrinology and Metab*, no. 10, October 1999: 837-41.

Isidori, A.M., et al. "Leptin and Androgens in Male Obesity: Evidence for Leptin Contribution to Reduced Androgen Levels," *J Clin Endocrinology and Metabolism* 84, no. 10 October 1999: 3673-80.

Kaplowitz, P. "Delayed Puberty in Obese Boys: Comparison with Constitutional Delayed Puberty and Response to Testosterone Therapy," *J of Pediatrics*, 133, no. 6 (December 1998):745-9.

Rosmond, R., and P. Björntorp. "Endocrine and Metabolic Aberrations in Men with Abdominal Obesity in Relation to Anxio-depressive Infirmity," *Metabolism* 47, no. 10 (October 1998):1187-93.

_____, and P. Björntorp. "The Interactions between Hypothalamic-Pituitary-Adrenal Axis Activity, Testosterone, Insulin-like Growth Factor I and Abdominal Obesity with Metabolism and Blood Pressure in Men," *Int J Obes Relat Metab Disord*, Dec 1998, 22, no. 12:1184-96.

Schöttner, M., et al. "Lignans from the Roots of Urtica dioica and Their Metabolites Bind to Human Sex Hormone Binding Globulin (SHBG)," *Planta Med*, Dec 1997, 63, no. 6: 529-32.

Shippen, E. and W. Fryer. *The Testosterone Syndrome: The Critical Factor for Energy, Health and Sexuality*, New York: M. Evans and Company, 1998.

Swartz, C. "Low Serum Testosterone: A Cardiovascular Risk in Elderly Men," *In Geriatric Med Today* 7, Dec 1998, no. 12.

Tchernof, A., et al. "Relationships between Endogenous Steroid Hormone, Sex Hormone-Binding Globulin and Lipoprotein Levels in Men: Contribution of Visceral Obesity, Insulin Levels and Other Metabolic Variables," *Atherosclerosis*, Sept 133, no. 2: 235-44.

Vermeulen, A., et al. "Testosterone, Body Composition and Aging," *J Endocrinol Invest*, 1999, 22, no. 5: 110-6.

Volek, J.S., et al. "Testoserone and Cortisol in Relationship to Dietary Nutrients and Resistance Exercise," *J of Applied Physiology* 82, no. 1 (January 1997): 49-54.

Wright, J. and L. Lenard. *Maximize Your Vitality & Potency: For Men over 40*, Petaluma, CA: Smart Publications, 1999.

CHAPTER 4

Backstrom, T. "Neuroendocrinology of Premenstrual Syndrome," *Clin Obset & Gynecol*, 35 (1992):612.

Barnes, S. "The Chemopreventive Properties of Soy Isoflavonoids in Animal Models of Breast Cancer," *Breast Cancer Res Treat*, Nov 1997, 46:2-3, 169-79.

_____ "Soy Isoflavonoids and Cancer Prevention. Underlying Biochemical and Pharmacological Issues," *Adv Exp Med Biol*, 401 (1996): 87-100.

Baumgartner, R.N., et al. "Associations of Fat and Muscle Masses with Bone Mineral in Elderly Men and Women," *Am J Clin Nutr*, 63: 365.

Bouchard, C., et al. "Inheritance of the Amount and Distribution of Human Body Fat," *Int J Obesity*, 1988, 12: 205.

Castleman, M. *The Healing Herbs*, New York: Bantam, 1995.

Cauley, J.A., et al. "The Epidemiology of Serum Sex Hormones in Postmenopausal Women," *Am J Epidem*, 1989, 129: 1120.

Ferraro, R., et al. "Lower Sedentary Metabolic Rates in Women Compared with Men," *J Clin Invest*, 1992, 90: 780.

Futagawa, N.K., et al. "Effect of Age on Body Composition and Resting Metabolic Rate," *Am J Physiol*, 1990, 259: E233.

Ingram, D., et al. "Case-Control Study of Phytoestrogens and Breast Cancer," *Lancet*, Oct 1997, 350: 990-94.

Journal of Nutrition, 2001, 131:1826-1832.

Kaym, S., et al. "Associations of Body Mass and Fat Distribution with Sex Hormone Concentrations in Postmenopausal Women," *Int J Epidemiol*, 1991, 151.

King, B.J. and M.A. Schmidt. *Bio-Age: Ten Steps to A Younger You*, Macmillan Canada, 2001.

Knudsen, C. "Super Soy: Health Benefits of Soy Protein," *Energy Times*, Feb 1996:12.

Laux, M. and C. Conrad. *Natural Woman, Natural Menopause*, New York: HarperCollins Inc., 1998.

Ley, C.J., et al. "Sex and Menopausal Associated Changes in Body Fat Distribution," *Am J Clin Nutr*, 1992, 55: 950.

Mauriège, P. et al. "Abdominal Fat Cell Lipolysis, Body Fat Distribution, and Metabolic Variables in Premenopausal Women," *J of Clin Endocrinology and Metab*, Oct 1990.

Messina, M.J., et al. Second International Symposium on the Role of Soy in Preventing and Treating Chronic Diseases, Brussels (September 19, 1996): 36.

Mindell, E. *Earl Mindell's Soy Miracle*, New York: Simon & Schuster, 1995.

Morgan, P., et al. *The Female Body: An Owners Manual: A Head to Toe Guide to Good Health and Body Care*, PA: Rodale Press Inc., 1996.

Pasquali, R., et al. "Body Weight, Fat Distribution and the Menopausal Status in Women," *Int J Obesity*, 1994, 18, no. 9: 614-21.

Rink, J.D., et al. "Cellular Characterization of Adipose Tissue from Various Body Sites of Women," *J of Clin Endocrinology and Metab*, July 1996.

Simpson, E. "Regulation of Estrogen Biosynthesis by Human Adipose Cells," *Endocrin Rev*, 1989, 10: 136.

Walker, M. "Concentrated Soybean Phytochemicals," *Healthy & Natural Journal*, 1994, 2, no. 2.

_____"Phytochemicals in Soybeans," *Health Foods Business*, March 1995: 36.

Waterhouse, D. *Outsmarting the Midlife Fat Cell*, New York: Hyperion, 1998.

Zamboni, M., et al. "Body Fat Distribution in Pre and Post-menopausal Women: Metabolic and Antropometric Variables in the Interrelationships," *Int J Obesity*, 1992, 16: 495.

Zeligs, M.A. "Plant-Powered Weight Loss: Phytonutrition for a Fat Burning Metabolism," 2001.

CHAPTER 5

Bar Or, O., et al. "Physical Activity, Genetic, and Nutritional Considerations in Childhood Weight Management," *Med Sci Sports Exerc*, 1998, 30, no. 1: 2-10.

Bellizi, M.C. and W. H. Dietz. "Workshop on Childhood Obesity: Summary of the Discussion," *Am J of Clin Nutr* (1999 supplement), 70:173S-5S.

Birch, L.L. "Development of Food Acceptance Patterns in the First Years of Life," *Proc Nutr Soc*, 1998, 57, no. 4: 617-24.

Caprio, S. et al., "Metabolic Impact of Obesity in Childhood," *Endocrinol Metab Clin North Am*, 1999, 28, no. 4: 731-47.

Colgan, M. *Colgan Chronicles: So You Think Milk Is Good for You?*, Vol. 4, Nu. 4, 2001.

Cutting, T.M., et al. "Like Mother, Like Daughter: Familial Patterns of Overweight Are Mediated by Mothers' Dietary Disinhibition," *Am J Clin Nutr*, 1999, 69, no. 4: 608-13.

Dewey, K.G., et al. "Breast-Fed Infants Are Leaner Than Formula-Fed Infants at 1 Year of Age: The DARLING Study," *Am J Clin Nutr*, Feb 1993 57, no. 2: 140-45.

Ebbeling, C.B. and N.R. Rodriguez. "Effects of Exercise Combined with Diet Therapy on Protein Utilization in Obese Children," *Med Sci Sports Exerc*, 1999, 31, no. 3: 378-85.

Fallon, S. and M. Enig. "Tragedy and Hype, The Third International Soy Symposium," *Nexus Magazine*, Apr-May 2000, 7, no. 3.

Golan, M.I., et al. "Parents as the Exclusive Agents of Change in the Treatment of Childhood Obesity," *Am J Clin Nutr*, 1998, 67, no. 6: 1130-35.

Irvine, C., et al. "The Potential Adverse Effects of Soybean Phytoestrogens in Infant Feeding," *New Zealand Med J*, May 24, 1995: 318.

Keller, J.D., et al. "Infants of Diabetic Mothers with Accelerated Fetal Growth by Ultrasonography: Are They All Alike?" *Am J Obstet Gynec*, Sept 1990, 163, no. 3: 893-97.

Levy, J.R., et al. "The Effect of Prenatal Exposure to the Phytoestrogen Genestein on Sexual Differentiation in Rats," *Proc Soc Exp Biol Med*, Jan 1995, 208, no. 1: 60-6.

Metzger, B.E., et al. "Amniotic Fluid Insulin Concentration as a Predictor of Obesity," *Arch Dis Child*, Oct 1990, 65, no. 10: 1050-52.

Patel, M.S., et al. "Overview of Pup in a Cup Model: Hepatic Lipogenesis in Rats Artificially Reared on a High-Carbohydrate Formula," *J Nutr* (Feb 1993 supplement), 123, no. 3: 373-77.

"Proceedings of the Nutrition Society," 1992, 51: 353-65.

Robinson, T.N. "Does Television Cause Childhood Obesity?" *JAMA*, 1998, 279, no. 12: 959-60.

Rosenbloom, A.L., et al. "Emerging Epidemic of Type 2 Diabetes in Youth," *Diabetes Care*, 1999, 22, no. 2: 345-54.

Santti, R., et al. "Phytoestrogens: Potential Endocrine Disruptors in Males," *Toxicol Ind Health*, Jan 1998, 14: 1-2, 223-37.

Setchell, K.D., et al. "Isoflavone Content of Infant Formulas and the Metabolic Fate of These Early Phytoestrogens in Early Life," *Am J of Clin Nutr* (Dec 1998 supplement): 1453S-1461S.

Silverman, B.L., et al. "Long-Term Prospective Evaluation of Offspring of Diabetic Mothers," *Diabetes 40* (December 1991, Supplement 2):121-25.

Slyper, A.H. "Childhood Obesity, Adipose Tissue Distribution, and the Pediatric Practitioner," *Pediatrics*, 102, no. 1 (1998):E4.

Sothern, M.S., et al. "A Multidisciplinary Approach to the Treatment of Childhood Obesity," *Del Med J*, 71, no. 6 (1999): 255-61.

Story, M. "School-Based Approaches for Preventing and Treating Obesity," *Int J Obes Relat Metab Disord*, 23 (1999 supplement): S43-51.

Strauss, R. "Childhood Obesity," *Curr Probl Pediatr*, 1999, 29, no. 1: 1-29.

Tanner, L. "Overweight Kids Have Potentially Dangerous Inflammation," *C Health*, Jan 10, 2001.

Whitten, P.L., et al. "Phytoestrogen Influences on the Development of Behavior and Gonadotrophin Function," *Proc Soc Exp Biol Med*, Jan 1995, 208, no.1: 82-86.

PART II: INTRO

Bernstein, G.A., et al. "Caffeine Withdrawal and the Effect on Normal Children," in Scientific Proceedings 43rd Annual Meeting of the American Academy of Child and Adolescent Psychiatry, Philadelphia, Penn., 1997.

Cherniske, S. *Caffeine Blues*, New York, NY: Warner Books, Inc., 1998.

"Estimated Annual Production and Consumption of Soft Drinks," Soft Drink Association, Washington, DC, 1987.

Kirschmann, J.D. *Nutrition Almanac* 4th edition, McGraw-Hill Professional Publishing, 1996.

Tollefson, L. and R.J. Barnard. "Analysis of FDA Passive Surveillance Reports of Seizures Associated with Consumption of Aspertame," *Journal of the Amer Dietetic Assoc*, 92, No.5, May 1992, 598-601.

Voreacos, D. "Experts Tell Panel of Continued Concern Over Use of Aspartame," *Los Angeles Times*, Nov. 4, 1987, p.19.

"You Are What You Drink, Too," *Los Angeles Times*, Dec. 22, 1996, p. E-2.

CHAPTER 6

Baba, N.H., et al. "High Protein vs. High Carbohydrate Hypoenergetic Diet for the Treatment of Obese Hyperinsulinemic Subjects," *Int J Obes Relat Metab Disord*, 1999, 23(11): 1202-6.

Bonora, E., et al. "Impaired Glucose Tolerance, Type II Diabetes Mellitus and Carotid Atherosclerosis: Prospective Results from the Bruneck Study," *Diabetologia*, 2000, 43: 2, 156-64.

Clemens, L.H., et al. "The Effect of Eating Out on Quality of Diet in Premenopausal Women," *J Am Diet Assoc*, 1999, 99(4): 442-4.

Daly, J.W., et al. "Is Caffeine Addictive? The Most Widely Used Psychoactive Substance in the World Affects Same Parts of the Brain as Cocaine," *Lakartindningen*, 1998, 95 (51-52): 5878-83.

Drummond, S., et al. "A Critique of the Effects of Snacking on Body Weight Status," *Eur J Clin Nutr*, 50(12): 779-83, 1996.

Garg, A., et al. "Effects of Varying Carbohydrate Content of Diet in Patients with Non-insulin-dependent Diabetes Mellitus," *JAMA*, 1994, 271 (18): 1421-8.

Garrett, B.E. and R.R. Griffiths. "Physical Dependence Increases the Relative Reinforcing Effects of Caffeine Versus Placebo," *Psychopharmacology* (Berl), 1998, 139 (3): 195-202.

Golay, A., et al. "Weight-loss with Low or High Carbohydrate Diet?" *Int J Obes Relat Metab Disord*, 1996, 20 (12): 1067-72.

Grant, W.B. "Low-fat, High-sugar Diet and Lipoprotein Profiles," *Am J Clin Nutr*, 1999, 70 (6): 1111-2.

Griffiths, R.R., et al. "Low-dose Caffeine Physical Dependence in Humans," *J Pharmacol Exp Ther*, 1990, 255 (3): 1123-32.

Harnack, L., et al. "Soft Drink Consumption Among U.S. Children and Adolescents: Nutritional Consequences," *J Am Diet Assoc*, 1999 (4): 436-41.

Hughes, J.R. and K.L. Hale. "Behavioral Effects of Caffeine and Other Methylxanthines on Children," *Exp Clin Psychopharmacol*, 1998, 6(1): 87-95.

Jeppesen, J., et al. "Effects of Low-fat, High-carbohydrate Diets on Risk Factors for Ischemic Heart Disease in Postmenopausal Women," *Am J Clin Nutr*, 1997, 65(4): 1027-33.

Lavin, J.H., et al. "The Effect of Sucrose and Aspartame Sweetened Drinks on Energy Intake, Hunger, and Food Choice of Female, Moderately Restrained Eaters," *Int J Obes Relat Metab Disord*, 1997, 21(1): 37-42.

McCrory, M.A., et al. "Overeating in America. Association Between Restaurant Food Consumption and Body Fatness in Healthy Adult Men and Women Ages 19 to 80," *Obes Res*, 1999, 7(6): 564-71.

Miller, J.C. "Importance of Glycemic Index in Diabetes," *Am J Clin Nutr*, 1994, 59: 747S-752S.

Reaven, G.M. "Do High Carbohydrate Diets Prevent the Development or Attenuate the Manifestations (Or Both) of Syndrome X? A Viewpoint Strongly Against," *Curr Opin Lipidol*, 1997, 8(1): 23-7.

Reaven, G.M. and C. Hollenbeck. "Variation of Insulin Stimulated Glucose Uptake in Healthy Individuals with Normal Glucose Tolerance," *J Clin Endocrinol Metab*, 1987, 64: 1169-1173.

Sidossis, L.S., et al. "Glucose Plus Insulin Regulates Fat Oxidation by Controlling the Rate of Fatty Acid Entry into the Mitochondria," *J Clin Invest*, 1996, 98 10: 2244-50.

Starc, T.J., et al. "Greater Dietary Intake of Simple Carbohydrate Is Associated with Lower Concentrations of High-Density-Lipoprotein Cholesterol in Hypercholesterolemic Children," *Am J Clin Nutr*, 1998, 67(6): 1147-54.

Strain, E.C., et al. "Caffeine Dependence Syndrome. Evidence from Case Histories and Experimental Evaluations," *JAMA*, 1994, 272(13): 1065-6.

Suga A., et al. "Effects of Fructose and Glucose on Plasma Leptin, Insulin, and Insulin Resistance in Lean and VMH-lesioned Obese Rats," *Am J Physiol Endocrinol Metab*, 2000, 278: 4, E677-83.

Wolfe, B.M. and L.A. Piche. "Replacement of Carbohydrate by Protein in a Conventional-fat Diet Reduces Cholesterol and Triglyceride Concentrations in Healthy Normolipidemic Subjects," *Clin Invest Med*, 1999, 22(4): 140-8.

CHAPTER 7

Barrsch, H., et al. "Dietary Polyunsaturated Fatty Acids and Cancers of the Breast and Colorectum: Emerging Evidence for Their Role as Risk Modifiers," *Carcinogenesis*, 1999, 20(12): 2209-18.

Berry, E.M. "Dietary Fatty Acids in the Management of Diabetes Mellitus," *Am J Clin Nutr*, 1997, 66 (4 Suppl): 991S-997S.

Blankson H, et al. "Conjugated Linoleic Acid Reduces Body Fat Mass in Overweight and Obese Humans," *J Nutr* 2000 Dec: 130(12):2943-8.

Bonnefont, J.P., et al. "Carnitine Palmitoyltransferase Deficiencies," *Mol Genet Metab*, 1999, 68(4): 424-40.

Borkman, M., et al. "The Relationship Between Insulin Sensitivity and the Fatty-Acid Composition of Skeletal-Muscle Phospholipids," *N Engl J Med*, 328(4): 238-44, 1993.

Broadhurst, C.L. "Balanced Intakes of Natural Triglycerides for Optimum Nutrition: An Evolutionary and Phytochemical Perspective," *Med Hypotheses*, 1997, 49(3): 247-61.

Cesano, A., et al. "Opposite Effects of Linoleic Acid and Conjugated Linoleic Acid on Human Prostatic Cancer in SCID Mice," *Anticancer Res*, 18 (3A): 1429-34, 1998.

Demmelmair, H., et al. "Trans Fatty Acid Contents in Spreads and Cold Cuts Usually Consumed by Children," *Z Ernahrungswiss*, 1996, 35(3): 235-40.

Dreon, D.M., et al. "A Very Low-Fat Diet Is Not Associated with Improved Lipoprotein Profiles in Men with a Predominance of Large, Low-density Lipoproteins," *Am J Clin Nutr*, 1999, 69 (3): 411-8.

Garg, A. "High-Monounsaturated-Fat Diets for Patients with Diabetes Mellitus: A Meta-analysis," *Am J Clin Nutr*, 1998, 67(3 Suppl): 577S-582S.

Gittleman, A.L. *The 40-30-30 Phenomenon*, Connecticut: Keats Publishing Inc., 1997.

Harris, W.S., et al. "Influence of n-3 Fatty Acid Supplementation on the Endogenous Activities of Plasma Lipase," *Am J Clin Nutr*, 1997, 66 (2): 254-60.

Heleniak, E. and B. Aston. "Prostaglandins, Brown Fat and Weight Loss," *Med Hypoth*, 1989, 28:13-33.

Horrocks, L.A. and Y.K. Yeo. "Health Benefits of Docosahexaenoic Acid (DHA)," *Pharmacol Res*, 1999, 40 (3): 211-25.

Ip, C. "Review of the Effects of Trans Fatty Acids, Oleic Acid, N-3 Polyunsaturated Fatty Acids, and Conjugated Linoleic Acid on Mammary Carcinogenesis in Animals," *Am J Clin Nutr*, 1997, 66 (6 Suppl): 1523S-1529S.

King, B.J. and M.A. Schmidt. *Bio-Age: Ten Steps to A Younger You*, Macmillan Canada, 2001.

Kwiterovich, P.O., Jr. "The Effect of Dietary Fat, Antioxidants, and Pro-Oxidants on Blood Lipids, Lipoproteins, and Atherosclerosis," *J Am Diet Assoc*, 1997 (7 Suppl): S31-41.

Lardinois, C.K. "The Role of Omega-3 Fatty Acids on Insulin Secretion and Insulin Sensitivity," *Med Hypotheses*, 1987, 24 (3): 243-8.

Louheranta, A.M., et al. "A High-Trans Fatty Acid Diet and Insulin Sensitivity in Young Healthy Women," *Metabolism*, 1999, 48 (7): 870-5.

Madsen, L., et al. "Eicosapentaenoic and Docosahexaenoic Acid Affect Mitochondrial and Peroxisomal Fatty Acid Oxidation in Relation to Substrate Preference," *Lipids*, 1999, 34 (9): 951-63.

Mori, T.A., et al. "Dietary Fish as a Major Component of a Weight-Loss Diet: Effect on Serum Lipids, Glucose, and Insulin Metabolism in Overweight Hypertensive Subjects," *Am J Clin Nutr*, 1999 70(5): 817-25.

Nelson, G.J., P.C. Schmidt, and D.S. Kelly. "Low-fat Diets Do Not Lower Plasma Cholesterol Levels in Healthy Men Compared to High-fat Diets with Similar Fatty Acid Composition at Constant Calorie Intake," *Lipids*, 1995, 30(11): 969-76.

Phinney, S.D. "Arachadonic Acid Maldistribution in Obesity," *Lipids*, 1996, 31 Suppl: S271-4.

Phinney, S.D. "Metabolism of Exogenous and Endogenous Arachidonic Acid in Cancer," *Adv Exp Med Biol*, 1996, 399: 87-94.

Rieger, M.A., et al. "A Diet High in Fat and Meat but Low in Dietary Fibre Increases the Genotoxic Potential of Ofecal Water 1," *Carcinogenesis*, 1999, 20 (12): 2311-6.

Riserus, U., et al. "Conjugated Linoleic Acid (CLA) Reduced Abdominal Adipose Tissue in Obese Middle-aged Men with Signs of the Metabolic Syndrome: A Randomized Controlled Trial," *Int J Obes Relat Metab Disord* 2001, Aug: 25(8):1129-35.

Rustan, A.C., et al. "Omega-3 and Omega-6 Fatty Acids in the Insulin Resistance Syndrome," *Ann NY Acad Sci*, 1997, 20 (827): 310-26.

Schlundt, D. "Randomized Evaluation of a Low-Fat Diet for Weight Reduction," *Int J Obesity*, 1993, 17: 623-9.

Schmidt, M.A. *Smart Fats*, Berkeley, Cal.: North Atlantic Books, 1997.

Sears, B. *The Anti-Aging Zone*, New York, NY: HarperCollins, Inc., 1999.

Simoneau, J.A., et al. "Markers of Capacity to Utilize Fatty Acids in Human Skeletal Muscle: Relation to Insulin Resistance and Obesity and Effects of Weight Loss," *FASEB J*, 1999, 13(14): 2051-60.

Simopoulos, A.P. "Is Insulin Resistance Influenced by Dietary Linoleic Acid and Trans Fatty Acids?" *Free Radic Biol Med*, 1994, 17(4): 367-72.

Tutelian, V.A., et al. "Effects of Polyunsaturated Fatty Acids of the Omega-3 Family in the Anti-Atherosclerotic Diet on the Activity of Lysosomal Lipolytic Enzymes, Mononuclear Cells and Blood Platelets of Patients with Ischemic Heart Disease," *Vopr Pitan*, 1993 (5): 17-2.

Willett, W.C., et al. "Is Dietary Fat a Major Determinant of Body Fat?" *Am J Clin Nutr*, 1998, 67: 556S-562S.

Willumsen, N., et al. "Eicosapentaenoic Acid, but Not Docosahexaenoic Acid, Increases Mitochondrial Fatty Acid Oxidation and Upregulates 2,4-Dienoyl-Coa Reductase Gene Expression in Rats," *Lipids*, 1996, 31(6): 579-92.

CHAPTER 8

Barenys, M., et al. "Effect of Exercise and Protein Intake on Energy Expenditure in Adolescents," *Rev Esp Fisiol*, 1993, 49(4): 209-17.

Biolo, G., et al. "An Abundant Supply of Amino-Acids Enhances the Metabolic Effect of Exercise on Muscle Protein," *Amer J Phys*, 1997, 273: E122-E129.

Bounous, G., et al. "Evolutionary Traits in Human Milk Proteins," *Med Hypotheses*, Oct 1998, 27: 2, 133-40.

Bounous, G., et al. "The Immunoenhancing Property of Dietary Whey Protein Concentrate," *Clin Invest Med*, Aug 1988, 11: 4, 271-8.

Bounous, G., et al. "The Influence of Dietary Whey Protein on Tissue Glutathione and the Diseases of Aging," *Clin Invest Med*, Dec 1989, 12: 6, 343-9.

Bounous, G., G. Batist and P. Gold. "Whey Proteins in Cancer Prevention," *Cancer Lett*, May 1999, 57: 2, 91-4.

Bounous, G. and P. Gold. "The Biological Activity of Undenatured Dietary Whey Proteins: Role of Glutathione," *Clin Invest Med*, Aug 1991, 14: 4, 296-309.

Campbell, W.W., et al. "Effects of an Omnivorous Diet Compared with a Lactoovovegetarian Diet on Resistance-Training-Induced Changes in Body Composition and Skeletal Muscle in Older Men," *Am J Clin Nutr*, 1999, 70: 1032-9.

Cassidy, C.M. "Nutrition and Health in Agriculturalists and Hunter-Gatherers: A Case Study of Two Prehistoric Populations," *Nutr Anth:* Pleasantville, New York: Pedgrave: 117-145.

Chaitow, L. *Amino Acids in Therapy,* Thorsons Publishers Inc., Rochester, VT, 1985.

Conley, E. *America Exhausted,* Flint, MI: Vitality Press Inc, 1998.

Coyne, L.L. *Fat Won't Make You Fat,* Alberta: Fish Creek Publishing, 1998.

Demonty, I., et al. "Dietary Proteins Modulate the Effects of Fish Oil on Triglycerides in the Rat," *Lipids,* 1998, 33(9): 913-21.

Froyland, L., et al. "Mitochondrion Is the Principal Target for Nutritional and Pharmacological Control of Triglyceride Metabolism," *J Lipid Res,* 1997, 38 (9): 1851-8.

Heine, W., et al. "Alpha-Lactalbumin-Enriched Low-Protein Infant Formulas: A Comparison to Breast Milk Feeding," *Acta Paediatr,* 1996, Sept, 85 (9): 1024-8.

Knudsen, C. "Super Soy: Health Benefits of Soy Protein," *Energy Times,* Feb, 1996: 12.

Lemon, P.W., et al. "Moderate Physical Activity Can Increase Dietary Protein Needs," *Can J Appl Physiol,* 1997, 22 (5): 494-503.

Longcope, C., et al. "Diet and Sex Hormone-Binding Globulin," *J Clin Endocrinol Metab,* 2000, 85: 1, 293-6.

McCarty, M.F. "Vegan Proteins May Reduce Risk of Cancer, Obesity, and Cardiovascular Disease by Promoting Increased Glucagon Activity," *Med Hypotheses,* 1999, 53 (6): 459-85.

Mindell, E. *Earl Mindell's Soy Miracle,* Simon & Schuster, 1995.

Morr, C.V. and E.Y. Ha. "Whey Protein Concentrates and Isolates: Processing and Functional Properties," *Crit Rev Food Sci Nutr,* 1993, 33: 6, 431-76.

Rankin, J.W. "Role of Protein in Exercise," *Clin Sports Med,* 18(3): 499-511, 1999.

Robinson, S.M., et al. "Protein Turnover and Thermogenesis in Response to High-Protein and High-Carbohydrate Feeding in Men," *Am J Clin Nutr,* 1990, 52 (1): 72-80.

Satterlee, L.D,. et al. "In Vitro Assay for Predicting Protein Efficiency Ratio as Measured by Rat Bioassay: Collaborative Study," *J Assoc Off Anal Chem,* Jul 1982, 65: 4, 798-809.

Soucy, J. and J. Leblanc. "Protein Meals and Postprandial Thermogenesis," *Physiol Behav,* 1999, 65 (4-5).

Stroescu, V., et al. "Effects of Supro Brand Isolated Soy Protein Supplement in Male and Female Elite Rowers," *XXVth FIMS World Congress of Sports Medicine,* Athens, Greece, 1994.

Vandewater, K. and Z. Vickers. "Higher-Protein Foods Produce Greater Sensory-Specific Satiety," *Physiol Behav,* 1996, 59(3): 579-83.

Walker, M. "Concentrated Soybean Phytochemicals," *Healthy & Natural Journal,* 1994, Vol.2, No.2.

Walker, M. "Phytochemicals in Soybeans," *Health Foods Business,* March 1995: 36.

Westerterp, K.R., et al. "Diet Induced Thermogenesis Measured over 24h in a Respiration Chamber: Effect of Diet Composition," *Int J Obes Relat Metab Disord,* 1999, 23 (3): 287-92.

Whitehead, J.M., et al. "The Effect of Protein Intake on 24-Hour Energy Expenditure During Energy Restriction," *Int J Obes Relat Metab Disord,* 1996, 20(8): 727-32.

Wurtman, J.J. and S.Suffers. *The Serotonin Solution,* Ballantine Books, 1997.

Zed, C. and W.P. James. "Dietary Thermogenesis in Obesity. Response to Carbohydrate and Protein Meals: The Effect of Beta-Adrenergic Blockage and Semi-Starvation," *Int J Obes,* 10 (5): 391-405, 1986.

CHAPTER 9

Baumel, S. *Serotonin: How to Naturally Harness the Power Behind Prozac and Phen/Fen.,* Keats Publishing, 1997.

Birdsall, T.C. "Hydroxytryptophan: A Clinically-Effective Serotonin Precursor," *Altern Med Rev,* Aug 1998, 3, no. 4: 271-80.

Bolla, K.I., et al. "Memory Impairment in Abstinent MDMA ("Ecstasy") Users," *Neurology,* Dec 1998, 51, no. 6: 1532-37.

Dye, L. and J.E. Blundell. "Menstrual Cycle and Appetite Control: Implications for Weight Regulation," *Hum Reprod,* June 1997, 12, no. 6: 1142-51.

Heine, W., et al. "Alpha-Lactalbumin-Enriched Low-Protein Infant Formulas: A Comparison to Breast Milk Feeding," *Acta Paediatr,* Sept 1996, 85, no. 9: 1024-28.

Knudsen, C. "Super Soy: Health Benefits of Soy Protein," *Energy Times,* Feb 1996: 12.

Leibowitz, S. and T. Kim. "Impact of a Galanin Antagonist on Exogenous Galanin and Natural Patterns of Fat Ingestion," *Brain Research,* 1992, 599: 148-52.

Leibowitz, S., et al. "Insulin Plays Role in Controlling Fat Craving," *News from The Rockefeller University,* New York, NY, 1995.

Morr, C.V. and E.Y. Ha. "Whey Protein Concentrates and Isolates: Processing and Functional Properties," *Crit Rev Fod Sci Nutr,* 1993, 33, no. 6: 431-76.

Prasad, C. "Food, Mood and Health: A Neurobiologic Outlook," *Braz J Med Biol Res,* Dec 1998, 31, no. 12: 1517-27.

Somer, E. and N.L. Snyderman. *Food & Mood: The Complete Guide to Eating Well and Feeling Your Best,* Owl Books, 1999.

Toornvliet, A.C., et al. "Serotoninergic Drug-Induced Weight Loss in Carbohydrate Craving Obese Patients," *Int J Obes Relat Meb Disord,* Oct 1996, 20, no. 10: 917-20.

Wiley, T.S. and B. Formby. *Lights Out: Sleep, Sugar, and Survival,* New York: Simon & Schuster, Inc., 2000.

Wurtman, J.J. "Carbohydrate Craving: Relationship Between Carbohydrate Intake and Disorders of Mood," *Drugs,* 39 (Supplement 3, 1990): 49-52.

Wurtman, J.J. and S. Suffers. *The Serotonin Solution,* New York: Ballantine Books, 1997.

Wurtman, R.J., et al. "Brain Serotonin, Carbohydrate-Craving, Obesity and Depression," *Adv Exp Med Biol,* 398, 1996. 35-41.

CHAPTER 10

Colgan, M. *Optimum Sports Nutrition,* New York: Advanced Research Press, 1993.

Colgan, M. *The New Nutrition: Medicine for the Millennium,* Apple Publishing, 1995, 153-54.

Colmers, W., et al. "Integration of NPY, AGRP, and Melanocortin Signals in the Hypothalamic Paraventricular Nucleus: Evidence of a Cellular Basis for the Adipostat," *Neuron,* 1999, 24: 155-163.

Conley, E. *America Exhausted,* Michigan: Vitality Press, 1998.

Germano, C. *Advantra Z: The Natural Way to Lose Weight Safely,* Kensington Publishing Corp., 1998.

King, B.J. and M.A. Schmidt. *Bio-Age: Ten Steps to A Younger You,* Macmillan Canada, 2001.

Klein, S. "The War against Obesity: Attacking a New Front," *Am J Clin Nutr,* June 1999, 69(6): 1061-1063.

Lowenstein, N.J. "Effect of Hydroxy-Citrate on Fatty Acid Synthesis by Rat Liver in Vivo," *J Biol Chem,* 1971, 246:629-632.

Markert, D. *The Turbo-Protein Diet,* BioMed International, 1999.

McGarry, J.D., et al, "Role of Carnitine in Hepatic Ketogenesis," *Proc Natl Acad Sci,* 1995, 72: 4385-4388.

McGarry, J.D. and D.W. Foster. "Regulation of Hepatic Fatty Acid Production and Ketone Body Production," *Ann Rev Biochem,* 1980, 49: 395-420.

Rosenfeld, R.D., et al. "Biochemical, Biophysical, and Pharmacological Characterization of Bacterially Expressed Human Agouti-Related Protein," *Biochemistry*, Nov 1998, 37: 46, 16041-52.

Sapolsky, R. *Why Zebras Don't Get Ulcers*, New York: W.H. Freeman and Company, 1998.

CHAPTER 11

Ahlborg, G. and P. Felig. "Influence of Glucose Ingestion on Fuel-Hormone Response During Prolonged Exercise," *J Appl Physiol*, 1976, 41: 683.

Biolo, G., et al. "An Abundant Supply of Amino Acids Enhances the Metabolic Effect of Exercise on Muscle Protein," *Amer J Physiol*, 1997, 273: E122-E129.

Blom, P.C.S., et al. "Effect of Different Post-Exercise Sugar Diets on the Rate of Muscle Glycogen Synthesis," *Med & Sci in Sports & Exercise*, 1987, 19: 491-496.

Burke, E.R. *Optimal Muscle Recovery*, New York: Avery Publishing Group, 1999.

D'Adama, P.J. *Eat Right for Your Type*, New York: Putnam, 1996.

Noakes, T.D. et al. "The Metabolic Response to Squash Including the Influence of Pre-Exercise Carbohydrate Ingestion," *S Afr Med J*, Nov. 1982, 62:20, 721-3.

CHAPTER 12

Chromium

Anderson, R.A. "Effects of Chromium on Body Composition and Weight Loss," *Nutr Rev* 1998: 56(9): 266-70.

Grant, K.E., et al. "Chromium and Exercise Training: Effect on Obese Women," *Med Sci Sports Exerc*, 1997, 29, no. 8: 992-98.

Kaats, G.R., et al. "A Randomized, Double-Masked, Placebo-Controlled Study of the Effects of Chromium Picolinate Supplementation on Body Composition: A Replication and Extension of a Previous Study," *Curr Ther Res*, 1998, 59: 379-88.

Vincent, J.B. "Mechanisms of Chromium Action: Low-Molecular-Weight Chromium-Binding Substance," *J Am Coll Nutr*, 1999, 18, no. 1: 6-12.

Citrus Aurantium

Astrup, A., et al. "Pharmacology of Thermogenic Drugs," *Am J Clin Nutr*, 1992.

Berry, M., et al. "The Contribution of Hepatic Metabolism to Diet-Induced Thermogenesis," *Metabolism*, 1985, 34: 141-47.

Collins, S., et al. "Strain Specific Response to Beta-3 Adrenergic Receptor Agonist Treatment of Diet Induced Obesity in Mice," *Endocrinol*, 1997, 138: 405-13.

Fleury, C., et al. "Uncoupling Protein-2: A Novel Gene Linked to Obesity and Hyper-insulinemia," *Nat Genetics*, 1997, 15: 269-72.

Gurley, B.J., et al. "Ephedrine Pharmacokinetics after the Ingestion of Nutritional Supplements Containing Ephedra Since (Ma Huang)," *Ther Drug Monit*, 1998, 4: 439-45.

Kaats, G. "Effects of Multiple Herbal Formulation on Body Composition, Blood, Chemistry, Vital Signs and Self-Reported Energy Levels and Appetite Control," *Int J Obesity*, 1994.

Mersmann, H. "Evidence of Classic Beta-3 Adrenergic Receptors in Porcine Adipocytes," *J Anim Sci*, May 1996, 74, no. 5: 984-92.

Yang, Y., et al. "Multiple Actions of Beta Adrenergic Agonists on Skeletal Muscle and Adipose Tissue," *Biochem J*, 1989.

Craving Formulas

Abraham, G.E. "Nutritional Factors in the Aetiology of the Premenstrual Tension Syndromes," *J Reprod Med* 1983, 28(7): 446-64.

Blum, K., et al. "Reward Deficiency Syndrome: A Biogenetic Model for the Diagnosis and Treatment of Impulsive, Addictive, and Compulsive Behaviors," *J Psychoactive Drugs* 2000, 32: Suppl: i-iv, 1-112.

Blum, K., et al. "The D2 Dopamine Receptor Gene as a Determinant of Reward Deficiency Syndrome," *J R Soc Med* 1996, 89(7): 396-400.

Bruinsma, K. and D.L. Taren. "Chocolate: Food or Drug?" *J Am Diet Assoc*, 99(10): 1249-56.

Cangiano, C., et al. "Eating Behavior and Adherence to Dietary Prescriptions in Obese Adult Subjects Treated with 5-hydroxytryptophan," *Am J Clin Nutr* 1992, 56: 863-7.

Cangiano, C., et al. "Effects of Oral 5-hydroxytryptophan on Energy Intake and Macro-nutrient Selection in Non-insulin-dependent Diabetic Patients" *Int J Obes Relat Metab Disord* 1998, 22(7): 648-54.

Ceci, F., et al. "The Effects of Oral 5-hydroxytryptophan Administration on Feeding Behavior in Obese Adult Female Subjects," *J Neural Transm* 1989, 76(2): 109-17.

Comings, D.E. and K. Blum. "Reward Deficiency Syndrome: Genetic Aspects of Behavioural Disorders," *Prog Brain Res* 2000, 126: 325-41.

Jiao, D.H., et al. "Clinical Study on Rhubarb Extract Tablet in Treating Simple Obesity," *Chin J Integr Tradit West Med* 2001, 7: 33-5.

Kelly, G.S. "Rhodiola Rosea: A Possible Plant Adaptogen," *Altern Med Rev* 2001, 6(3): 293-302.

Wang, G.J., et al. "Brain Dopamine and Obesity," *Lancet* 2001, 357(9257): 354-7.

Wurtman, R.J. and J.J. Wurtman. "Brain Serotonin, Carbohydrate-craving, Obesity and Depression," *Adv Exp Med Biol* 196, 398: 35-41.

EFAs

Harris, W.S., et al. "Influence of n-3 Fatty Acid Supplementation on the Endogenous Activities of Plasma Lipase," *Am J of Clin Nut*, 1997, 66, no. 2: 254-60.

Madsen, L., et al. "Eicosapentaenoic and Docosahexaenoic Acid Affect Mitochondrial and Peroxisomal Fatty Acid Oxidation in Relation to Substrate Preference," *Lipids*, 1999, 34, no. 9: 951-63.

Schmidt, M.A. *Smart Fats*, Berkeley: North Atlantic Books, 1997.

Simoneau, J.A., et al. "Markers of Capacity to Utilize Fatty Acids in Human Skeletal Muscle: Relation to Insulin Resistance and Obesity and Effects of Weight Loss," *FASEB J*, 1999, 13, no. 14: 2051-60.

Willett, W.C., et al. "Is Dietary Fat a Major Determinant of Body Fat?" *Am J Clin Nutr*, 1998, 67: 556S-562S.

Forskolin

Ahmad, F., et al. "Insulin and Glucagon Releasing Activity of Coleonol (Forskolin) and Its Effects on Blood Glucose Level in Normal and Alloxan Diabetic Rats," *Acta Diabetol Lat*, Jan 1991, 28, no. 1: 71-77.

Metzger, H., and E. Lindner. "The Positive Inotropic-Acting Forskolin, a Potent Adenylate Cyclase Activator," *Arzneimittelforschung*, 1981, 31, no. 8: 1248-50.

Murray, M. "The Unique Pharmacology of Coleus Forskohlii," *Health Counselor*, no. 2.

Seamon, K. "Structure-Activity Relationships for Activation of Adenylate Cyclase by the Diterpene Forskolin and Its Derivatives," *J Med Chem*, March 1983, 26, no. 3: 436-39.

Green Food Concentrate
Colgan, M., and L. Colgan. *The Flavonoid Revolution*, Vancouver: Apple Publishing, 1997.
Graci, S. *The Power of Superfoods: 30 Days That Will Change Your Life*, Toronto: Prentice Hall Canada, Inc., 1997.

Green Tea
Deng, Z., et al. "Effect of Green Tea and Black Tea on Blood Glucose, Triglycerides, and Antioxidants in Aged Rats," *J Agricult Food Chem*, 1998, 46: 3875-78.
Dulloo, A. "Efficacy of a Green Tea Extract Rich in Catechin Polyphenols and Caffeine in Increasing 24h. Energy Expenditure and Fat Oxidation in Humans," *Am J of Clin Nut*, 1999, 70: 1040-45.
Hara, Y. "Influence of Tea Catechins on the Digestive Tract," *J Cel Biochem.*
Yokogoshi, H., et al. "Effect of Theanine, R-Glutamylethylamide, on Brain Monoamines and Striatal Dopamine Release in Conscious Rats," *Neurochem Res*, 1998, 46: 2143-50.

Hydroxycitric Acid
Lowenstein, N. "Effect of Hydroxycitrate on Fatty Acid Synthesis by Rat Liver in Vitro," *J Biol Chem*, 1971.
McGarry, J., and D. Foster. "Regulation of Hepatic Fatty Acid Production and Ketone Body Production," *Ann Rev Biochem*, 1980, Novin, D. et al. *Am J Clin Nutr*, 1985, 42: 1050-62.
Sullivan, A. *Am J Clin Nutr*, 30 1977: 767-76.

L-carnitine
Clouet, P., et al. "Effect of Short- and Long-Term Treatments by a Low Level Dietary L-carnitine on Parameters Related to Fatty Acid Oxidation in Winstar Rat," *Biochem Biophys Acta*, 1996, 1299, no. 2: 191-97.
McGarry, J.D. "More Direct Evidence for a Malonyl-CoA-Carnitine Palmitoyltransferase I Interaction as a Key Event in Pancreatic Beta-Cell Signaling," *Diabetes*, 1994, 43: 878-83.
Paulson, D.J. "Carnitine Deficiency-Induced Cardiomyopathy," *Mol Cell Biochem*, 1998, 180: 33-41.
Reyes, B., et al. "Effects of L-carnitine on Erythrocyte Acyl-CoA, Free CoA, and Glycerophospholipid Acyltransferase in Uremia," *Am J of Clin Nut*, 1998, 67, no. 3: 386-90.
Rubaltelli, F.F., et al. "Carnitine & the Premature Biol Neonate."

Protein Isolate
Bounous, G. and P. Gold. "The Biological Activity of Undenatured Dietary Whey Proteins: Role of Glutathione," *Clin Invest Med*, Aug 1991, 14: 296-309.
Knudsen, C. "Super Soy: Health Benefits of Soy Protein," *Energy Times*, Feb 1996: 12.
Life Extension Foundation (The). *The Wonders of Whey: Restoring Youthful Anabolic Metabolism at the Cellular Level*, May 1999.
Mindell, E. *Earl Mindell's Soy Miracle*, New York: Simon & Schuster, 1995.
Renner, E. *Milk and Dairy Products in Human Nutrition*, Munich, 1983.
Volpi, E., et al. "Exogenous Amino Acides Stimulate Net Muscle Protein Synthesis in the Elderly," *Clin Invest*, 1998, 101: 2000-07.
Walker, M. "Concentrated Soybean Phytochemicals," *Healthy & Natural Journal*, 1994 2, no. 2.
_____. "Phytochemicals in Soybeans, Health," *Foods Business*, March 1995: 36.

Supplement Antioxidant

Bounous, G. and P. Gold. "The Biological Activity of Undenatured Dietary Whey Proteins: Role of Glutathione," *Clin Invest Med*, 1991 Aug, 14:4, 296-309.

Colgan, M. *Antioxidants, The Real Story*, Apple Publishing Co. Ltd., 1998.

Conley, E.J. *America Exhausted: Breakthrough Treatments of Fatigue and Fibromyalgia*, Vitality Press Inc, 1997.

Gy, J.Y., et al. "Effects of Sesamin and Alpha-tocopherol, Individually or in Combination on the Polyunsaturated Fatty Acid Metabolism, Chemical Mediator Production, and Immunoglobulin in Sprague-Dawley Rats," *Biosci Biotechnol Biochem*, 59(12): 2198-202, 1995.

Kagan, T., et al. "Coenzyme Q10 Can in Some Circumstances Block Apoptosis, and This Effect Is Mediated Through Mitochondria," *Ann NY Acad Sci*, 887: 31-47, 1999.

Kishi, Y., et al. "Alpha-lipoic Acid: Effect on Glucose Uptake, Sorbitol Pathway, and Energy Metabolism in Experimental Diabetic Neuropathy," *Diabetes*, 48(10): 2045-51, 1999.

Krinsky, N.I., et al. "Antioxidant Vitamins and Beta-carotene in Disease Prevention," *Am J Clin Nutr*, 6(S): 1299S-1540S, 1995.

Lang, I., et al. "Effect of the Natural Bioflavonoid Antioxidant Silymarin on Superoxide Dismutase (SOD) Activity and Expression in Vitro," *Biotachnol Ther*, 4: 263-70, 1993.

Packer, L., and C. Colman. *The Antioxidant Miracle*, John Wiley & Sons, 1999.

Pressman, A.H. *Glutathione, The Ultimate Antioxidant*, The Philip Lief Group, Inc, 1997.

Sinatra, S.T. *The Coenzyme Q10 Phenomenon*, Keats Publishing, 1998.

Streeper, R.S., et al. "Differential Effects of Lipoic Acid Stereoisomers on Glucose Metabolism in Insulin-resistant Skeletal Muscle," *Am J Physiol*, 273(1 Pt 1): E185-91, 1997.

CHAPTER 13

Andrews, J.F. "Exercise for Slimming," *Proc Nutr Soc* Aug 1991, 50, no. 2: 459-71.

Borsheim, E., et al. "Adrenergic Control of Post-Exercise Metabolism," *Acta Physiol Scand*, March 1998, 162, no. 3: 313-23.

Brynr, R.W., et al. "Effects of Resistance vs. Aerobic Training Combined with an 800 Calorie Liquid Diet on Lean Body Mass and Resting Metabolic Rate," *J Am Coll Nutr*, 1999, 18, no. 2: 115-21.

Burke, E.R. *Optimal Muscle Recovery*, New York: Avery Publishing Group, 1999.

Carlson, L.A., et al. "Studies on Blood Lipids During Exercise," *J Lab Clin Med* 1963, 61: 724-29.

Chilibeck, P.D., et al. "Higher Mitochondrial Fatty Acid Oxidation Following Intermittent versus Continuous Endurance Exercise Training," *Can J Physiol Pharmacol*, Sept 1998, 76, no. 9: 891-94.

Coggan, A.R. et al. "Fat Metabolism During High-Intensity Exercise in Endurance-Trained and Untrained Men," *Metabolism*, 2000, 49, no. 1: 122-28.

Colgan, M. *The New Nutrition*, Chapter 25, Vancouver: Apple Publishing, 1995.

Esmarck B., J.L. Andersen, S. Olsen and M.M. Richter. "Timing of Post-exercise Protein Intake Is Important for Muscle Hypertrophy with Resistance Training in Elderly Humans," *Journal of Physiology*, 535:301-311, 2001.

Felig, P. and F. Wahren. "Fuel Homeostasis in Exercise," *NE J Med*, 1975, 293:1078-1084.

Fernández, Pastor V.J., et al. "Function of Growth Hormone in the Human Energy Continuum During Physical Exertion," *Rev Esp Fisiol*, Dec 1991, 47, no. 4: 223-29.

Herring, J.L., et al. "Effect of Suspending Exercise Training on Resting Metabolic Rate in Women," *Med Sci Sports Exerc*, Jan 1992, 24, no. 1: 59-65.

Hunter, G.R., et al. "A Role for High-Intensity Exercise on Energy Balance and Weight Control," *Int J Obes Relat Metab Disord*, 1998, 22, no. 6: 489-93.

Kraemer, W.J. et al. "Effects of Heavy-Resistance Training on Hormonal Response Patterns in Younger and Older Men," *J Appl Physiol*, 1999, 87, no. 3: 982-92.

McCartney, N.A., et al. "Usefulness of Weightlifting Training in Improving Strength and Maximal Power Output in Coronary Artery Disease," *Amer J Cardiol*, 1991, 67: 939.

Muller, W.A., et al. "The Influence of the Antecedent Diet upon Glucagon and Insulin Secretion," *NE J Med*, 1971, 285:1450-1454.

Pavlou, K.N., et al. "Effects of Dieting and Exercise on Lean Body Mass, Oxygen Uptake and Strength," *Med Sci Sports Exer*, 1985, 17: 466-71.

Poehlman, E.T. "A Review: Exercise and Its Influence on Resting Energy Metabolism in Man," *Med Sci Sports Exerc*, Oct 1989, 21, no. 5: 515-25.

Sears, B. *The Anti-Aging Zone*, New York: Regan Books, 1999.

van Dale, D., et al. "Weight Maintenance and Resting Metabolic Rate 18-40 Months After a Diet/Exercise Treatment," *Int J Obes*, April 1990, 14, no. 4: 347-59.

CHAPTER 14

Batmanghelidj, F. *Your Body's Many Cries for Water*, Falls Church, VA: Global Health Solutions, 1998.

Burke, E.R. *Optimal Muscle Recovery*, Garden City Park, NY: Avery Publishing Group, 1999.

Fleck, S.J. and W.J. Kraemer. *Periodization Breakthrough*, New York: Advanced Research Press, 1996.

Index